MILITARY AND VETERAN ISSUES

TREATMENT OF PTSD AND TRAUMATIC BRAIN INJURY AMONG VETERANS

Military and Veteran Issues

Additional books in this series can be found on Nova's website
under the Series tab.

Additional E-books in this series can be found on Nova's website
under the E-book tab.

Neurology - Laboratory and Clinical Research Developments

Additional books in this series can be found on Nova's website
under the Series tab.

Additional E-books in this series can be found on Nova's website
under the E-book tab.

MILITARY AND VETERAN ISSUES

TREATMENT OF PTSD AND TRAUMATIC BRAIN INJURY AMONG VETERANS

AIDEN D. THOMAS
AND
MILTON L. HARRIS
EDITORS

nova publishers

Nova Science Publishers, Inc.
New York

For permission to use material from this book please contact us:
Telephone 631-231-7269; Fax 631-231-8175
Web Site: http://www.novapublishers.com

Additional color graphics may be available in the e-book version of this book.

Library of Congress Cataloging-in-Publication Data

ISBN: 978-1-62081-689-9

Published by Nova Science Publishers, Inc. ✢ New York

CONTENTS

PREFACE

Two combat-related conditions that affect some veterans who have served in Iraq and Afghanistan and that have generated widespread concern among policymakers are post-traumatic stress disorder (PTSD), and traumatic brain injury (TBI). This book explores the clinical care that the Veterans Health Administration (VHA), the health care system within the Department of Veterans Affairs, provides for recent combat veterans; VHA's coordination with the Department of Defense for the care of service members returning from Iraq and Afghanistan; the prevalence of PTSD and TBI among veterans of those conflicts and the occurrence of those conditions among recent combat veterans using VHA's services; and the costs to VHA of providing care and management to recent combat veterans for these conditions.

Chapter 1 - More than 2 million service members have deployed in support of overseas contingency operations (OCO) in Iraq and Afghanistan since October 2001. Some military service members receive medical care in the combat theater for injuries or other medical conditions sustained while deployed. Other service members have combat-related medical conditions that are identified and treated after they return from war—within the Department of Defense's (DoD's) health care system for active-duty personnel and within the Department of Veterans Affairs (VA) for veterans, including deactivated reservists. VA provides health care services through the Veterans Health Administration (VHA), which treats veterans for service-connected conditions and other conditions.

VHA spent about $2 billion (in 2011 dollars) in fiscal year 2010 to treat veterans of recent overseas contingency operations, compared with total expenditures in 2010 on health care for veterans of all eras and conflicts of about $48 billion. From 2002 through 2010, VHA spent a total of $6 billion on health care expenditures for recent OCO veterans.

Chapter 2 - Traumatic brain injury (TBI) has emerged as a serious concern among U.S. forces serving in military operations in Afghanistan and Iraq. The widespread use of improvised explosive devices in these conflicts increases the likelihood that servicemembers will sustain a TBI, which the Department of Defense (DOD) defines as a traumatically induced structural injury and/or physiological disruption of brain function as a result of an external force. TBI cases within DOD are generally classified as mild, moderate, severe, or penetrating. From 2000 to March 2011 there were a total of 212,742 TBI cases reported by the Defense and Veterans Brain Injury Center within DOD. A majority of these cases, 163,181, were classified as mild traumatic brain injuries (mTBI)—commonly referred to as concussions.

Early detection of injury is critical in TBI patient management. Diagnosis of moderate and severe TBI usually occurs in a timely manner due to the obvious and visible nature of the head injury. Identification of mTBI presents a challenge due to its less obvious nature. With mTBI, there may be no observable head injury. In addition, in the combat theater, an mTBI may not be identified if it occurs at the same time as other combat injuries that are more visible or life-threatening, such as orthopedic injuries or open wounds. Furthermore, some of the symptoms of mTBI—such as irritability and insomnia—are similar to those associated with other conditions, such as post-traumatic stress disorder.

Chapter 3 - The Clinical Practice Guideline for the Management of Concussion/Mild Traumatic Brain Injury (mTBI) was developed under the auspices of the Veterans Health Administration (VHA) and the Department of Defense (DoD) pursuant to directives from the Department of Veterans Affairs (VA). VHA and DoD define clinical practice guidelines as:

"Recommendations for the performance or exclusion of specific procedures or services derived through a rigorous methodological approach that includes:

- Determination of appropriate criteria such as effectiveness, efficacy, population benefit, or patient satisfaction; and
- Literature review to determine the strength of the evidence in relation to these criteria."

The intent of these guidelines is to:

- Reduce current practice variation and provide facilities with a structured framework to help improve patient outcomes
- Provide evidence-based recommendations to assist providers and their patients in the decision-making process related to the patient health care problems
- Identify outcome measures to support the development of practice-based evidence that can ultimately be used to improve clinical guidelines.

In: Treatment of PTSD and Traumatic Brain Injury ... ISBN: 978-1-62081-689-9
Editors: Aiden D. Thomas and Milton L. Harris

Chapter 1

THE VETERANS HEALTH ADMINISTRATION'S TREATMENT OF PTSD AND TRAUMATIC BRAIN INJURY AMONG RECENT COMBAT VETERANS*

Congress of the United States
Congressional Budget Office

NOTES

Unless otherwise indicated, all years referred to in this study are federal fiscal years (which run from October 1 to September 30).

Unless otherwise indicated, all dollar amounts in this study are expressed in 2011 dollars. Before providing cost data to the Congressional Budget Office (CBO), the Veterans Health Administration converted those data to fiscal year 2009 dollars on the basis of annual increases in the average cost of a primary care visit from 2004 to 2009. CBO indexed those data to 2011 dollars using the implicit price deflator for gross domestic product. CBO also converted other dollar amounts reported in this study to 2011 dollars using the implicit price deflator for gross domestic product.

Numbers in the text and tables may not add up to totals because of rounding.

PREFACE

Two combat-related conditions that affect some veterans who have served in Iraq and Afghanistan and that have generated widespread concern among policymakers are post-traumatic stress disorder (PTSD) and traumatic brain injury (TBI). In response to a request from the Ranking Member of the House Committee on Veterans' Affairs, this Congressional Budget Office (CBO) study examines the following:

---

* This is an edited, reformatted and augmented version of Congress of the United States, Congressional Budget Office, dated February 2012.

- The clinical care that the Veterans Health Administration (VHA), the health care system within the Department of Veterans Affairs, provides for recent combat veterans;
- VHA's coordination with the Department of Defense for the care of service members returning from Iraq and Afghanistan;
- The prevalence of PTSD and TBI among veterans of those conflicts and the occurrence of those conditions among recent combat veterans using VHA's services; and
- The costs to VHA of providing care to recent combat veterans for those conditions.

In keeping with CBO's mandate to provide objective, impartial analysis, this study makes no recommendations.

Elizabeth Bass and Heidi Golding of CBO's National Security Division prepared the study under the general supervision of David Mosher and Matthew Goldberg. Allison Percy served as the internal reviewer. Lindsay Coleman, Juan Contreras, Sunita D'Monte, and Ann Futrell provided thoughtful comments on a draft of the study, as did external reviewer Rajeev Ramchand of RAND Corporation. (The assistance of an external reviewer implies no responsibility for the final product, which rests solely with CBO.) Adebayo Adedeji fact-checked the manuscript. The authors wish to thank the Department of Veterans Affairs and the Department of Defense for providing data used in the analysis.

Juyne Linger edited the study, and John Skeen proofread it. Cindy Cleveland produced drafts of the manuscript. Maureen Costantino prepared the paper for publication and designed the cover. Monte Ruffin printed the initial copies, and Linda Schimmel handled the print distribution.

Douglas W. Elmendorf
Director

SUMMARY

More than 2 million service members have deployed in support of overseas contingency operations (OCO) in Iraq and Afghanistan since October 2001. Some military service members receive medical care in the combat theater for injuries or other medical conditions sustained while deployed. Other service members have combat-related medical conditions that are identified and treated after they return from war—within the Department of Defense's (DoD's) health care system for active-duty personnel and within the Department of Veterans Affairs (VA) for veterans, including deactivated reservists. VA provides health care services through the Veterans Health Administration (VHA), which treats veterans for service-connected conditions and other conditions.

VHA spent about $2 billion (in 2011 dollars) in fiscal year 2010 to treat veterans of recent overseas contingency operations, compared with total expenditures in 2010 on health care for veterans of all eras and conflicts of about $48 billion. From 2002 through 2010, VHA spent a total of $6 billion on health care expenditures for recent OCO veterans.

Two conditions that affect some military service members during deployment to a combat theater and afterward are post-traumatic stress disorder (PTSD) and traumatic brain injury (TBI). PTSD is an anxiety disorder induced by exposure to a traumatic event, such as witnessing injury or death. It is characterized by symptoms that include reexperiencing the event, hyperarousal (irritability, anger, or hypervigilance, for example), and diminished responsiveness to or avoidance of stimuli associated with the trauma.

TBI is caused by sudden trauma to the head and is commonly sustained by soldiers exposed to explosions. It may result in a decreased level of consciousness, amnesia, or neurological abnormalities, and it is classified as mild, moderate, or severe on the basis of its severity at the time of the injury. Mild TBI, which is also known as a concussion, may in some cases lead to ongoing symptoms that include headaches, memory difficulties, fatigue, irritability, and sleep problems. Diagnosing severe cases is straightforward, but mild TBIs—which account for about 90 percent of TBI cases among active-duty OCO service members—may be difficult to detect, both by those afflicted and by health care professionals, although most cases resolve quickly without medical intervention.[1]

Summary Table 1. The First Year of Treatment for All Health Care Provided to OCO Patients by VHA

Treatment Group	Average Cost per Patient (Dollars)	Number of OCO Patients	Share of All OCO Patients (Percent)
PTSD or TBI			
PTSDa	8,300	103,500	21
TBI[b]	11,700	8,700	2
Both PTSD and TBI	13,800	26,600	5
No PTSD or TBI	2,400	358,000	72
Polytrauma	136,000	500	*

Source: Congressional Budget Office based on data from the Department of Veterans Affairs, Veterans Health Administration.

Notes: Data cover fiscal years 2004 to 2009 for the first year of treatment.

All of the TBI patients in the data that CBO examined had symptomatic TBI—that is, they exhibited symptoms that were attributed to TBI at the time of VHA's medical screening or examination.

VHA converted costs provided to CBO to fiscal year 2009 dollars on the basis of annual increases in the average cost of a primary care visit from 2004 to 2009. CBO then indexed those costs to 2011 dollars using the implicit price deflator for gross domestic product.

OCO = overseas contingency operations; VHA = Veterans Health Administration; PTSD = post-traumatic stress disorder; TBI = traumatic brain injury; * = less than 1 percent.

[a] Patients in the PTSD group did not have TBI, but many had other conditions.

[b] Patients in the TBI group did not have PTSD, but many had other conditions.

Some observers contend that DoD and VHA may not adequately screen, diagnose, and treat OCO service members and veterans affected by PTSD and mild TBI. In this study, the Congressional Budget Office (CBO) analyzes VHA's care of OCO patients diagnosed with PTSD or TBI and compares the reported rates of occurrence of those conditions within VHA with estimates of the prevalence of those conditions in the broader population of service members who have deployed to recent overseas contingency operations. (Prevalence estimates gauge the proportion of cases of a disease or condition in a population, whether or not people have received a diagnosis from a medical professional; by comparison, the reported occurrence of conditions among the people who have been treated within VHA reflects counts of diagnoses by medical professionals.) The study also examines the costs that VHA has incurred in treating patients diagnosed with PTSD and TBI.

In brief, CBO finds:

- Among OCO patients treated by VHA from 2004 through 2009, 21 percent were diagnosed with PTSD (but not TBI) and 2 percent with symptomatic TBI (but not PTSD) (see Summary Table 1).[2] An additional 5 percent had both PTSD and TBI; thus, about 75 percent of those diagnosed with TBI had a concurrent diagnosis of PTSD. Seventy-two percent of patients had neither diagnosis. (CBO separately analyzed another 500 polytrauma patients—that is, ones with complex, severe injuries to multiple organ systems.)
- The average cost for OCO patients in the first year of their treatment was about four to six times greater for patients with a diagnosis of PTSD, TBI, or both than for patients without those conditions.
- VHA's average costs for OCO patients were highest during the first year of care and generally declined and then stabilized in subsequent years.
- For patients with TBI (including those with both PTSD and TBI), however, VHA's average treatment costs appear to increase in the third and fourth years of care. That result is probably driven by a policy change that occurred in the middle of the period that CBO analyzed and the nature of the data that VHA provided to CBO.[3] In the absence of the policy change, costs for those patients probably also would have been highest during the first year of care and then declined and stabilized thereafter.
- A great deal of uncertainty surrounds the prevalence of PTSD and TBI within the OCO population and, hence, the number of veterans with those conditions that DoD, VHA, and other health care providers may encounter in the future.

Projecting the future costs of treating veterans with PTSD and TBI requires estimating both the number of patients with those conditions who will seek VHA's care and the costs per patient that VHA will incur. Because the research community has not reached a consensus about the prevalence of those conditions, such projections would be highly uncertain. CBO examined published studies that reported the prevalence of PTSD or TBI among different groups of service members or veterans who had deployed to overseas contingency operations. For PTSD, those prevalence estimates have generally ranged between 5 percent and 25 percent. For TBI, those estimates indicate that between 15 percent and 23 percent of service members may have experienced a TBI while deployed to an overseas contingency operation but that a smaller share, between 4 percent and 9 percent, are still symptomatic when screened after returning to the United States. Estimates of the prevalence of PTSD and TBI vary widely among studies because of substantial differences in the assessment tools that researchers use to identify the conditions, the stringency of the criteria they employ, and the subgroups they sample. The percentage of OCO veterans whom VHA clinicians have diagnosed with PTSD (26 percent) is at the top of the range reported in published studies, whereas the percentage they have diagnosed with symptomatic TBI (7 percent) is in the middle of the reported range.

The rates of diagnosis of PTSD and TBI among OCO veterans seeking treatment at VHA do not necessarily reflect the prevalence of those conditions in the entire OCO population. If veterans who suspected they had mental health or other medical problems were more likely than other veterans to seek medical care from VHA, the rates of PTSD and TBI diagnosed among VHA's patients would tend to overestimate the prevalence in the entire OCO population. However, some veterans might not seek care from VHA for various reasons—the stigma associated with having a mental health problem, for example, or the inconvenience of undergoing additional evaluation and treatment. If a sufficient number of veterans with PTSD and TBI did not seek care from VHA, the rates of diagnoses for those conditions among VHA's patients would tend to underestimate the prevalence in the OCO population.

INTRODUCTION

The United States has been involved in overseas contingency operations (OCO) in Afghanistan and Iraq since October 2001 and March 2003, respectively, and has deployed more than 2 million service members in support of those operations. The Department of Defense (DoD) delivers medical care to service members while they are deployed. That care includes nearly 4 million medical encounters since January 2005 for a variety of conditions, including injuries; it also includes 71,000 medical evacuations of service members from the combat theaters through November 2011. Both DoD and the Veterans Health Administration (VHA), the organization that provides medical care within the Department of Veteran Affairs (VA), screen for various conditions and provide health care after service members return from deployment. VHA treated 400,000 (31 percent) of 1.3 million eligible OCO veterans in fiscal year 2010, up from 100,000 (20 percent) of 500,000 eligible OCO veterans in 2005. Many eligible veterans do not seek care at VHA in any given year or at any time, and most VHA patients seek additional health care outside of VHA. (See Box 1 for information about eligibility for VHA's health care system.) Although OCO veterans made up 7 percent of the patients VHA treated in 2010, they accounted for only 4 percent ($2 billion) of the $48 billion (in 2011 dollars) that VHA obligated for medical care that year. From 2002 through 2010, VHA spent a total of $6 billion on health care for OCO veterans.[4]

Two medical conditions that may affect OCO veterans have received particular attention: post-traumatic stress disorder (PTSD) and traumatic brain injury (TBI). PTSD is an anxiety disorder triggered by a traumatic event, such as may occur when engaging in combat; witnessing serious injury, brutality, or unnatural death, particularly of another soldier; or suffering a severe vehicle accident, including those caused by improvised explosive devices (IEDs). The symptoms of PTSD include reexperiencing the event, hyperarousal (irritability, anger, or hypervigilance, for example), and diminished responsiveness to or avoidance of stimuli associated with the trauma. TBI is a blow to the head that alters a person's consciousness, if only momentarily. TBI may result in amnesia or neurological abnormalities at the time of injury. In the combat theater, explosions from IEDs or other bombs are a leading cause of TBI among military personnel, although TBIs also result from falls, motor vehicle accidents, and bullet wounds.[5] TBI is classified as mild, moderate, or severe on the basis of its severity at the time of injury. (That classification refers to the acuteness of initial symptoms only, not to that of persistent symptoms.) Mild TBI, also known as a concussion, typically resolves quickly without medical treatment, in many cases within weeks and in most cases within three months. Although some symptoms may linger for six months or more, there is considerable debate over whether those persistent symptoms can be attributed to mild TBI or to other conditions.[6] (See Appendix A for more detailed information about PTSD and TBI.) Few service members have been evacuated from combat theaters as a result of PTSD or TBI alone, although many have been evacuated for TBI in conjunction with other injuries. Many cases of PTSD and TBI may go unrecognized and consequently undiagnosed and untreated, both in the combat theater and once the service member returns home. PTSD can interfere with daily functioning when it results in emotional withdrawal from family and friends, inappropriate expressions of anger, irritability, overprotective behaviors, or substance abuse. Those with ongoing mild TBI may feel sad, nervous, or agitated; have difficulty concentrating and sleeping; and experience sensitivity to noise or light. Those with moderate or severe TBI may experience similar difficulties but also have more complex physical and neurological limitations, which in some cases affect their ability to live independently. Symptoms manifest themselves in different ways and with different intensity across people and situations; some people function well in some settings but not in others.

Box 1. Eligibility for VHA's Services

Eligibility for the health care system of the Veterans Health Administration (VHA) is based primarily on a veteran's military service. Generally, veterans of the active components of the military must have served 24 continuous months on active duty to be eligible; reservists and National Guard members may be eligible if they are called to active duty under a federal order and they complete that service.

Those broad criteria, however, do not necessarily guarantee access to medical treatment. VHA operates an enrollment system that assigns a veteran to one of eight categories to establish his or her priority for using its health care services.

Veterans with higher priority include those who have service-connected disabilities, low income, or both. In January 2003, VHA imposed a general freeze (with some subsequent modifications) on new enrollments in the lowest priority group (Priority Group 8).[1]

The Veterans Programs Enhancement Act of 1998 (Public Law 105-368) guarantees access to VHA's health care system, after separation from active mili tary service, to members of the armed forces who have served on active duty in combat operations since the law was enacted in November 1998; reservists and members of the National Guard who have served in combat operations are also included under that guarantee.

The law gave combat veterans two years (starting from their date of separation from the military) to enroll and use VHA's health care system without requiring those veterans to document either that their income is below established thresholds or that they have a service-connected disability—requirements that noncombat veterans must fulfill.

In 2008, lawmakers extended the enhanced eligibility period for care through VHA's health care system to five years.[2]

Under those legislative authorities, VHA provides free health care for medical conditions directly or potentially related to a veteran's military service in combat operations for five years after separation.

Veterans who had deployed to overseas contingency operations (OCO) may continue to use VHA's services when the five-year period of enhanced eligibility ends, but their priority group for enrollment may change, depending on their disability status and income. In particular, OCO veterans may be moved to a lower priority group, including Priority Group 8, and incur the applicable copayments.

[1] Veterans in Priority Group 8 are those who have no service-connected disabilities (or, according to a determination by the Department of Veterans Affairs [VA], have service-connected disabilities that are ineligible for monetary compensation) and have annual income or net worth above VA's means-test threshold and regional income threshold. See www.va.gov/health eligibility/Library/AnnualThresholds.asp.

[2] See title XVII of the National Defense Authorization Act for Fiscal Year 2008, P.L. 110-181, 122 Stat. 493.

Some policymakers have questioned whether DoD and VHA have the resources and capacity to serve the OCO population with PTSD and TBI. Some observers are also concerned about whether service members and veterans with those conditions are reluctant to seek the help they need. In this study, the Congressional Budget Office (CBO) examines the clinical care provided by VHA for OCO veterans with PTSD and TBI, VHA's coordination with DoD for the care of service members and veterans, the rate of occurrence of PTSD and TBI among VHA patients and the estimated prevalence of those conditions in the broader population of recent OCO veterans, the use of VHA's health care services by OCO veterans who have been diagnosed with PTSD or TBI, and the costs of providing that care. Because the prevalence of PTSD and TBI in the OCO population is highly uncertain, CBO has not projected VHA's future costs for treating veterans with those conditions.

Clinical Care within VHA

To serve the growing population of veterans, VHA has hired more than 7,500 mental health professionals since 2005 and has established specialized rehabilitation centers for veterans with multiple complex injuries, including TBI. Further, VHA offers a broad range of services and programs tailored specifically to OCO patients with PTSD and TBI. In this section, CBO presents a brief overview of typical strategies for diagnosing PTSD and TBI, along with treatment options that VHA provides for those conditions.

VHA's Services for PTSD

As of September 2011, mental health diagnoses were the second largest diagnostic category among OCO veterans who had received health care services from VHA, affecting 52 percent of those patients.[7] VHA delivers PTSD care in primary care settings and in specialized programs of evaluation, treatment, and education. Through its electronic national clinical reminder system, VHA endeavors to administer a screening test for various medical conditions, known as the Iraq and Afghan Post-Deploy Screen, to all OCO patients.[8] That screen includes the Primary Care PTSD (PC-PTSD) screen, which consists of four questions.

VHA's policy is to screen for PTSD every year for the first five years a veteran uses VHA care and once every five years thereafter, except in cases in which a clinical need for more frequent screening has been identified.

Veterans who screen positive for PTSD are referred for additional evaluation. For most patients, further assessment is provided by a mental health professional such as a psychiatrist, psychologist, or trained clinician. That assessment typically takes place at a follow-up appointment, although additional evaluation or a diagnosis may occur during the visit when the screening occurs. VHA clinicians make their diagnoses according to the American Psychiatric Association's *Diagnostic and Statistical Manual of Mental Disorders* (DSM), which delineates the professionally certified criteria for mental disorders in the United States. Diagnoses are made using a variety of diagnostic tools, often in combination, such as structured interviews (the Clinician-Administered PTSD Scale), semistructured interviews (the Structured Clinical Interview for DSM Disorders), and self-reported evaluations (the PTSD Checklist).

Although PTSD has a well-validated case definition and diagnostic criteria, it can nonetheless be difficult to diagnose and treat. First, some OCO veterans and service members do not seek treatment for mental health problems. Despite widespread outreach programs within the military and VHA, the stigma associated with mental health disorders may discourage veterans from scheduling an appointment for an assessment or from requesting treatment, and fear of harming one's military career may inhibit service members from seeking treatment while they are on active duty. Second, as with many mental health disorders, there is no objective measure, such as a laboratory test result, for confirming a diagnosis of PTSD. Third, some PTSD symptoms—for example, irritability, emotional numbing, insomnia, and trouble concentrating—also occur with other conditions. Fourth, PTSD can impair judgment, especially if combined with associated conditions such as substance abuse, and thereby make it more difficult for veterans with PTSD to seek or maintain treatment.

VHA provides treatment for PTSD at VHA hospitals, outpatient clinics, community-based outpatient clinics (CBOCs), and Vet Centers.[9] In addition, VHA pays for some care delivered through outside providers. VHA reports that treatment for PTSD is commonly delivered in outpatient clinics and CBOCs, either through general mental health clinics or, less commonly, through specialized programs provided by PTSD Clinical Teams, Substance Use PTSD Teams, and Women's Stress Disorder Treatment Teams. VHA guidelines instruct clinicians to tell patients to expect about six months of treatment, but for patients with severe cases of PTSD or multiple diagnoses of mental health disorders, treatment may extend for one to two years or longer. For many veterans, PTSD oscillates between remission and relapse. The National Center for PTSD reports that some veterans may never be free of symptoms; rather, patients may learn coping mechanisms that allow them to function in private and public spheres. One of VHA's treatment goals is to help veterans develop those mechanisms.[10]

Treatment for PTSD is tailored to the patient and may include a combination of psychotherapy (treatment based on psychology techniques) and pharmacotherapy (treatment using prescription drugs). In addition, all treatment programs for PTSD in VHA provide education for families and veterans (including coping mechanisms).

VHA offers two forms of evidence-based psychotherapy—that is, therapy based on a substantive body of empirical research broadly accepted by the medical community. Those therapies are cognitive processing therapy (CPT) and prolonged exposure (PE) therapy. CPT helps patients change the way the trauma is perceived—for example, by replacing blame and guilt with less distressing thoughts. In PE therapy, the traumatic events are narrated repeatedly and combined with exercises to reduce anxiety in specific situations. The Institute of Medicine has concluded that exposure therapies, such as PE therapy, or other therapies that include exposure as part of treatment, such as CPT, are the only types of psychotherapy that have been found effective for PTSD; however, the Institute also noted evidence that the effectiveness of exposure therapies for veterans is not as strong as for civilians.[11] Other therapies used by VHA include group and family therapy.

Clinical research suggests that PTSD patients who undergo therapy require at least nine treatment sessions.[12] VHA reported to CBO that 40 percent of OCO veterans initiating CPT or PE therapy complete a full course of therapy. Typically, VHA patients undergoing CPT meet one on one with a therapist for an hour each week; for patients undergoing PE therapy, VHA typically schedules one 90-minute session each week. VHA data from internal program evaluations indicate that OCO veterans who completed PE therapy attended an average of 11 sessions, whereas those who did not complete therapy attended an average of 5 sessions; results were similar for patients undergoing CPT. Additional data from a recently published study found that 80 percent of OCO veterans who used VHA's services and received new PTSD diagnoses had at least one follow-up visit; nonetheless, fewer than half completed the recommended treatment sessions within one year.[13] The reasons for not completing a full course of therapy may include the following: the distance between home and the location of care, a preference for receiving mental health care from providers outside VHA, difficulty scheduling appointments, negative perceptions of mental health care, and impaired judgment as a result of either the condition itself or associated problems such as substance abuse.

Pharmacotherapy in VHA consists mainly of the use of antidepressants, such as selective serotonin reuptake inhibitors (SSRIs) and serotonin norepinephrine reuptake inhibitors (SNRIs). If unsuccessful, treatment may expand to mood stabilizers, anticonvulsants, antipsychotics, or other agents to alleviate symptoms such as anxiety, intrusive thoughts, flashbacks, and insomnia. In one study, VHA researchers determined that pharmacotherapy was more likely to be prescribed for patients receiving a diagnosis in a mental health clinic than for those diagnosed in a general medical or PSTD clinic.[14]

A small share of OCO patients with PTSD diagnoses undergoes psychiatric hospitalization—5 percent through 2010. Such hospitalizations include both traditional inpatient stays and specialized programs involving short residential stays; those stays involve counseling and treatment with social, vocational, and recreational therapies.

VHA's Services for TBI

TBI is classified as mild, moderate, or severe on the basis of its severity at the time of the injury. Because moderate and severe TBIs are easily identified and require immediate attention, acute care for combat-related TBIs is given by DoD, whereas VHA provides rehabilitation care. Moderate and severe TBIs are clinically different from mild TBIs, and their treatment typically involves substantially more health care resources. Veterans who experienced moderate or severe TBIs may receive inpatient rehabilitative care, outpatient rehabilitative care, or both, through programs that specialize in treating complex patients.

Along with occupational, cognitive, physical, and other therapies, VHA also provides advanced technologies to veterans with ongoing needs related to sensory impairment, communication deficits, mobility, and self-care. The course of treatment prescribed and the services provided vary significantly by patient and are tailored to the severity of the TBI and ongoing problems.

Veterans with mild TBI are also eligible for VHA's TBI rehabilitation programs, but they are usually treated on an outpatient basis for less intense clinical symptoms and for a much shorter duration than moderate and severe TBI patients. In April 2007, VHA directed that all OCO veterans who use VHA and have not received a prior diagnosis for TBI be screened for symptomatic TBI—that is, TBI with currently occurring symptoms such as headaches, memory difficulties, or sleep problems. Because moderate and severe cases are readily detected, the purpose of this screen, in effect, is to identify mild TBI. Since April 2007, questions designed to detect TBI have been included in VHA's Iraq and Afghan Post-Deploy Screen. For those who screen positive, additional evaluation takes place with the patient's agreement; in the absence of that consent, VHA requires that the patient's refusal to undergo further evaluation be documented. Through 2009, approximately one in five OCO veterans screened positive for symptomatic TBI. Two-thirds of those screening positive (or 14 percent of all screened patients) completed a comprehensive evaluation (some of those may not have undergone further testing because symptoms had resolved before the full evaluation was conducted). Of the 14 percent receiving a comprehensive evaluation, VHA clinicians diagnosed symptomatic TBI in one-half of those who screened positive (or 7 percent of all those initially screened).[15]

Some VHA medical facilities use individual neurologists, rehabilitation physicians, or psychiatrists for the follow-up evaluation, whereas others refer patients to an interdisciplinary team. Evaluation includes a complete history of injury, a physical exam, and a neurobehavioral inventory of TBI symptoms. Other diagnostic tools for TBI are limited. In some cases, a veteran's medical records from DoD are incomplete or unavailable, because DoD's and VHA's medical systems are not fully integrated. Correct diagnosis is problematic, as none of the symptoms of TBI are unique to that condition, and there is no clinically validated definition for TBI with persistent symptoms months after injury. Thus, many of the difficulties in diagnosing and treating PTSD also apply to symptomatic TBI: Some veterans may not seek care; there is no objective diagnostic tool to confirm the diagnosis; symptoms may coincide with those of other conditions; and VHA's diagnostic process often relies heavily on the veteran's memory, which may be impaired as a result of TBI or another medical condition.[16]

After confirmation of the diagnosis, additional physical examinations, laboratory tests, and psychosocial evaluations may be performed.[17] Because there is no standard treatment regimen, a team of clinicians typically evaluates the results and determines a treatment plan, which accounts for concurrent disorders.

According to VHA's guidelines, patients with symptoms persisting beyond four to six weeks of treatment should be reassessed, assigned to a case manager, and receive treatment for their remaining symptoms.

VHA considers the management of physical, behavioral, and cognitive symptoms fundamental to treatment of mild TBI. The two mainstays of treatment are symptom-specific treatment (such as managing headache pain, the most common symptom of TBI) and educating patients on their expected recovery. VHA states that treatment through primary care clinics is appropriate for managing TBI when implemented by an interdisciplinary team of rehabilitation therapists, pharmacists, and mental health clinicians. Pharmacotherapy is sometimes used alone or in conjunction with other therapies to treat musculoskeletal pain, anxiety, or psychiatric symptoms.

However, there is currently no clinically validated pharmacotherapy to improve neurocognitive function after a mild TBI. As with PTSD, providing education for veterans and families about TBI is an important part of treatment. VHA's guidelines advise providers to reassure patients and their families that mild TBI is normally transient and full recovery without permanent damage is expected.

Duration of treatment for mild TBI at VHA is normally one to three months, with follow-up four to six weeks later to confirm recovery, which is defined as the resolution of symptoms and normal functioning. For some patients, however, symptoms may persist beyond six months to a year or longer. Further evaluation for other conditions may be indicated for persistent symptoms.

Concurrent Diagnoses of PTSD and TBI

TBIs sustained in Iraq or Afghanistan are often the result of explosions and involve other injuries; moreover, PTSD has been shown to occur more commonly in veterans with combat-related concussions (mild TBIs) than in those with other injuries. The Institute of Medicine's Committee on Gulf War and Health found evidence, albeit limited, suggesting that TBI and PTSD are associated.[18] CBO's analysis of VHA data found that three-quarters of OCO patients with a TBI diagnosis also had a diagnosis of PTSD and that one-fifth of OCO patients with a PTSD diagnosis also had a diagnosis of TBI.[19]

Because PTSD and TBI may generate many of the same symptoms, a person who has both conditions may be diagnosed for only one and not the other or, alternatively, diagnosed with both but have only one condition. Medical consensus is lacking on the accuracy of screening and diagnosis for both conditions if the person has concurrent PTSD and TBI. Diagnosing only one of the conditions when both are present can lead to difficulties with treatments. For example, treatments for either mild TBI or PTSD alone may not be effective for patients with both conditions, as cognitive impairment may hinder adherence to treatment.

Polytrauma

VHA uses the designation "polytrauma" to describe complex, severe injuries to multiple organ systems that often result from the same event, such as an explosion. Those may include brain injury, amputation, hearing and vision impairments, spinal cord injuries, and psychological trauma. A small number of patients who have those complex injuries are treated in VHA's Polytrauma System of Care, which provides comprehensive, interdisciplinary rehabilitation and other care for seriously disabled patients. The Polytrauma System of Care includes five Polytrauma Rehabilitation Centers for inpatient rehabilitation, as well as secondary sites and clinical teams for postdischarge care.[20]

COOPERATION BETWEEN VHA AND DOD

Soon after the conflicts in Afghanistan and Iraq began, it became apparent that some wounded service members were encountering significant difficulties when making the transition from DoD's health care system to VHA's. To address those concerns, DoD and VHA have increased their cooperation and have devoted more resources to encouraging service members and veterans to seek care.[21]

In the summer of 2007, DoD and VHA instituted the Wounded, Ill, and Injured Senior Oversight Committee to address problems specific to those service members, which include the coordination of health care management, disability evaluation, and transition of OCO service members' health care from DoD to VHA.[22] The committee has several work groups charged with addressing particular issues, including one that focuses on the needs of service members and veterans with PTSD and TBI.

The Wounded Warrior Act, part of the National Defense Authorization Act for Fiscal Year 2008 (Public Law 110 181, sections 1601–1676) required DoD and VHA to implement many initiatives, including reducing waiting time for medical care, consolidating their disability evaluation systems, and establishing standards to determine whether and when wounded service members could return to active duty. The law also mandated that the Government Accountability Office (GAO) deliver progress reports on those initiatives to the Congress. In its July 2009 report, GAO found that although DoD and VHA had not fully developed or implemented the requirements of the Wounded Warrior Act, they had made considerable progress.[23]

DoD and VHA have targeted the coordination of health care management to service members with TBI or with PTSD and other mental health conditions. In particular, the agencies are collaborating on myriad issues such as screening, diagnosing, and treating those conditions, as well as assisting service members in their transition from DoD's health care system to that of VHA. One result of that collaboration is the TBI screen used by VHA, which was derived from the screen first used by DoD at certain military bases. DoD and VHA have formed joint committees, such as the VHA/DoD Mental Health Working Group; participate in joint research ventures, such as the Defense and Veterans Brain Injury Center; and share clinical practice guidelines, such as *Management of Concussion/Mild Traumatic Brain Injury*.[24] DoD and VHA clinicians may collaborate on service members' transition to VHA's care; however, the proliferation of programs and case managers can be confusing for service members and has led to some duplication of efforts.[25]

Because the sharing of medical records between DoD and VHA would greatly facilitate the transition of service members between the agencies, the Wounded Warrior Act included provisions designed to achieve such sharing; however, that objective remains a work in progress. DoD and VHA do have complex sharing agreements and information-exchange projects to coordinate their independent record systems. For example, DoD can transfer the medical records of service members who have separated from DoD and are eligible for VHA care through the Federal Health Information Exchange. Moreover, health care clinicians for DoD and VHA can access records for patients treated by providers in either agency through the Bidirectional Health Information Exchange. Yet technical and organizational challenges have made it difficult to construct a unified electronic medical record. The Virtual Lifetime Electronic Record (VLER)—a joint effort of DoD and VHA—overcame a major hurdle in

2010 when DoD and VHA agreed to use a common personal identifier. Slated for VHA-wide implementation in 2012, the VLER is a single electronic record that would be used to manage comprehensive administrative and medical information for service members throughout their lives, from enlistment to death, regardless of health care provider.

Current record-sharing goals for VHA and DoD extend to a broader effort with the private sector, the Nationwide Health Information Network (NwHIN)[26] This group of federal agencies and private organizations has agreed to securely share patients' health information electronically among providers and health care systems by defining standards, services, and policies. Pilot projects for NwHIN are under way; veterans who agree to participate allow their public- and private-sector health care providers to share specific health information.

CBO's Analytical Approach to VHA Data

In this study, CBO presents data on the use of VHA's health care services between fiscal years 2004 and 2009 by OCO veterans who received a diagnosis of PTSD or TBI.[27,28] CBO also presents estimates of the costs that VHA has incurred to treat OCO veterans with PTSD, TBI, or both during that period and compares them with the costs of providing care to OCO patients who do not have PTSD or TBI.[29] CBO's estimates are based on VHA's cost data and do not include expenditures by other federal providers of health care or private insurers, out-of-pocket costs, forgone earnings, or other losses to society associated with the two conditions.[30]

CBO's primary analysis focused on VHA patients who had not been treated at specialized polytrauma facilities, which provide care for veterans who suffer from more than one complex physical or mental trauma. That analysis examined the use of VHA's health care services and cost of providing those services for 496,800 OCO veterans in four mutually exclusive groups:

- 103,500 patients with PTSD (but not TBI);
- 8,700 patients with TBI (but not PTSD);
- 26,600 patients with both PTSD and TBI; and
- 358,000 patients with neither of those two conditions.[31]

Patients in the PTSD group did not have TBI, but many had other conditions; similarly, patients in the TBI group did not have PTSD, but many had other conditions. None of the groups includes 500 polytrauma patients, many with PTSD and TBI, who were analyzed separately. The data include 99 percent of all OCO veterans seen by VHA from 2004 to 2009. To protect patients' confidentiality, VHA did not provide CBO with data on individual patients. Because VHA did not identify the date of patients' first diagnosis or entry, CBO was not able to calculate the use or the cost of health care for patients entering VHA treatment in any given fiscal year.

For the first three groups, CBO presents data on the use of services and costs of treatment for the first year of care (treatment year 1) and for up to three additional years following initial diagnosis.[32] Data on patients with no diagnosis of PTSD or TBI are presented for comparison purposes following their initial visit for any VHA care. CBO did not receive detailed clinical data and thus was not able to construct a comparison group that was similar in all observed ways to the three groups apart from their diagnosis of PTSD, TBI, or both. The patients with and without PTSD or TBI were roughly similar in age, sex, and military experience, but they differed in certain characteristics, particularly injuries sustained while deployed in overseas contingency operations. In general, service members who had PTSD or TBI were more likely to have received other injuries, so the costs of care for the PTSD and TBI groups probably would have been higher even without the costs of care for PTSD and TBI. The poly-trauma group, which consisted of patients with multiple complex injuries requiring extended inpatient stays for rehabilitation at VHA, is examined separately later in the study; it was a very small group whose average medical costs were far higher than those of the four other groups.

CBO's analysis is based on data from VHA's administrative records from 2004 through 2009. Because some patients started using VHA's services partway through the sample period, not all patients were observed for the full six years. Indeed, CBO used only the first four years of data even when six years were available because data for that longer span existed for only a small minority of veterans. When fewer than four years of data existed, CBO included all of the years available. Consequently, when CBO examined patients' first year of treatment, those who entered the VHA system in 2008 and 2009 were included, but when CBO examined later years of treatment, those patients were not included, having entered the system too late in the sample period.

Not only do patients entering VHA in 2008 and 2009 have fewer years of treatment data available, they are also different from those who entered in earlier years in two other ways. First, more veterans entering the VHA system in those later years had experienced longer deployments and multiple deployments. Second, starting in 2008, VHA extended enhanced eligibility from two years to five years for OCO veterans (see Box 1 on page 2). That extension enabled veterans with delayed-onset PTSD or other combat-related conditions for which they had not previously sought treatment to enter the VHA system and receive care at no cost. However, CBO does not believe that those two differences substantially affected the number or severity of PTSD or TBI cases or, more generally, the injuries or other medical conditions treated at VHA in 2008 and 2009.[33]

While screening and treatment for PTSD were consistent across the years, VHA's clinical practices for TBI changed during the data period (2004 to 2009): The agency initiated comprehensive screening for mild, symptomatic TBI in 2007. As a consequence, the characteristics of TBI patients are likely to be different across treatment years. Patients whom VHA diagnosed with TBI before 2007 were more likely to have had moderate to severe TBI than those diagnosed in 2007 or after. The study period ended before the newly identified mild cases could accumulate four treatment years. Therefore, moderate and severe cases are more common among TBI patients in treatment years 3 and 4 than in treatment years 1 and 2. Because CBO did not have information on TBI severity (mild, moderate, or severe), it was not possible to separate the use of services and costs by severity. The costs of treating mild TBI, however, are likely to be substantially lower than the costs of treating moderate and severe TBI. As a result of the policy change, use and costs in later treatment years grow for TBI patients and are almost as high in treatment year 4 as in treatment year 1. Without the policy change, use and costs for those patients probably would have been highest during the first year of care and then declined and stabilized thereafter, as occurred in the other groups.

VHA provided CBO with aggregate use and cost data for groups of OCO veterans based on their demographic characteristics, medical condition, and medical services used.[34] Because data were provided at the group level, CBO can only present information on averages for those groups and not on the distribution of use or cost within groups. (For additional information about the data and methodology used in this analysis, see Appendix B.)

CBO calculated total and average costs for patients who accessed VHA's services at least once, for up to four years after their PTSD or TBI diagnoses or, in the absence of those diagnoses, average costs for up to four years after their entry into the VHA system. Diagnostic tests and pharmacy use were included and categorized as part of outpatient costs. As with all analyses based on administrative data, errors and nonstandardized coding may affect the results presented here.

OCCURRENCE AND PREVALENCE OF PTSD AND TBI

In the VHA data provided to CBO regarding 496,800 OCO veterans treated by VHA between 2004 and 2009, veterans with a diagnosis of PTSD (but not TBI) accounted for 21 percent (103,500) of the total, and those with a diagnosis of TBI (but not PTSD) accounted for 2 percent (8,700). In addition, veterans with diagnoses of both PTSD and TBI accounted for about 5 percent (26,600). Thus, three out of four OCO veterans with a diagnosis of TBI had a concurrent PTSD diagnosis.[35] In total, approximately 26 percent (130,100) had at least one diagnosis of PTSD, and 7 percent (35,300) had at least one diagnosis of TBI.[36] More than 70 percent (358,000) of OCO veterans treated by VHA were not diagnosed with either PTSD or TBI. Other mental health conditions besides PTSD are common within the OCO veteran population. (For a brief description of other mental health conditions and suicide in that population, see Box 2.)

The occurrence of PTSD and TBI among OCO veterans who use the VHA system—which is measured by the diagnosis rates just described—does not necessarily reflect the prevalence of those conditions in the entire OCO population. If service members who have separated from the military are more likely to have service-connected health problems than those who have remained on active duty, then the rate of diagnosis among VHA patients will be higher than the proportion of the entire OCO population that has those problems. If, however, sufficient numbers of veterans with PTSD or TBI were either being treated for the condition elsewhere or not being treated at all, the rate in the overall OCO population could be greater than the rate diagnosed among VHA patients. For example, some veterans have employment-based health insurance; others seek care from other sources that are not connected to their military service, perhaps because providers are located more conveniently or are perceived to be more private; and still other veterans forgo care altogether. For PTSD, the effect of stigma associated with a positive screening or diagnosis has not been measured well, but it is likely to reduce the number of people who admit to problems associated with PTSD and then screen positive. For those reasons, the prevalence—that is, the estimate of the proportion of cases in a population, whether or not the individual has received a clinical diagnosis from a medical professional—of PTSD and TBI in the OCO population probably differs from the percentage of patients in the VHA system diagnosed with those conditions.

Many researchers have estimated PTSD and TBI prevalence among different groups of service members and veterans who deployed to operations in Iraq and Afghanistan, but there is no consensus as to the prevalence rate among the entire OCO population.[37] Researchers generally have reported prevalence rates ranging between 5 percent and 25 percent for PTSD among different groups of service members who deployed to overseas contingency operations, with generally higher rates in studies of infantry brigades or combat teams. Researchers have found that the proportion of service members who experienced a TBI, including those who no longer had symptoms, ranged from 15 percent to 23 percent, and that the proportion of service members who had symptomatic TBI after returning from deployment ranged from 4 percent to 9 percent. Thus, the percentage of OCO veterans whom VHA clinicians have diagnosed with PTSD (26 percent) is at the top of the range of prevalence reported in published studies, whereas the percentage they have diagnosed with symptomatic TBI (7 percent) is in the middle of the reported range. The estimates of symptomatic TBI remain uncertain because there are no clinically validated diagnostic criteria for that condition, and connecting self-reported persistent symptoms to the initial injury is problematic. Published estimates of PTSD and TBI during deployment vary widely because the assessment tools used to identify the conditions, the criteria used to identify cases, and the subgroup of service members sampled differ among studies. (For a detailed discussion of those issues, see Appendix C.)

The gold standard for determining prevalence would be to evaluate each person in a representative sample of the OCO population using validated clinical interviews; achieving that ideal, however, would be expensive and difficult. Instead, some researchers use administrative data on diagnoses to measure the number of cases of PTSD and TBI; others use clinical screening tools to assess cases. Administrative data on diagnoses understate prevalence in a population because not everyone seeks care. Some researchers who use screening tools to identify PTSD and TBI apply low thresholds for assessing those conditions. In so doing, however, they may also generate many false positives and overestimate the number of cases. Conversely, researchers employing more restrictive thresholds could underestimate cases. In addition, most studies to date, including some that attempt to be population-based, have oversampled certain groups; applying rates from nonrandom samples without the proper weighting is unlikely to yield an accurate measurement of prevalence. On the one hand, estimates based on combat units, which experience higher rates of physical and psychological trauma than other types of military units, may lead to prevalence estimates that are too high to apply to the general population of service personnel in a combat region, which includes support units. On the other hand, samples based on returning, uninjured troops may lead to estimated prevalence rates that are too low.

Another shortcoming with published studies, which applies also to diagnosis rates within VHA, is that service members and veterans may not accurately report their symptoms. The stigma associated with screening positive for PTSD, the perceived inconvenience of undergoing additional evaluation, or a lack of confidence in treatment effectiveness may lead to an underreporting of symptoms of mental health problems or TBI and thus an underestimate of prevalence. Finally, using estimates of TBIs that occur during deployment is problematic because even a confirmed clinical diagnosis when or shortly after an injury is sustained does not reveal the frequency of persistent postconcussive symptoms. DoD reports that, although a small minority of service members has ongoing symptoms, most cases of TBI are mild, often resolving within weeks and almost always improving within three months.

USE OF VHA'S SERVICES

Through September 2011, VHA reported that the number of OCO veterans who had used VHA at least once totaled nearly 740,000, or 53 percent of OCO veterans. The OCO population using VHA's services tends to be male (88 percent), is young (46 percent are younger than 32), consists predominantly of former soldiers in the Army (61 percent), and is slightly more likely to be veterans of active-duty units (56 percent) than reserve components.

Future spending on OCO patients will change according to the mix of conditions diagnosed and the number of patients treated.[38] CBO's estimates of diagnosis rates are useful in projecting VHA's future costs, but the usefulness depends on the extent to which the prevalence of those conditions and veterans' likelihood to seek treatment at VHA remain the same. If outreach services motivate more veterans to seek care, for example, the rate at which veterans use VHA's services would tend to increase over time. Combat exposure should decline with OCO troop levels, however, so fewer service members are likely to develop PTSD or TBI in the future. In addition, an increasing share of veterans who do seek care from VHA in the future will have deployed several years earlier and are more likely to have sought care through DoD or to have had their symptoms resolve than was the case for veterans who sought care from VHA before 2010. For those reasons, future veterans enrolling in VHA's health care system are less likely to seek treatment for PTSD or TBI.

Box 2. Suicide and Mental Illness among OCO Veterans

Just over half of veterans of overseas contingency operations (OCO) treated by the Veterans Health Administration (VHA) have a diagnosis of a mental illness. Mental health problems can affect all aspects of life. Suicide among service members and veterans, an infrequent but devastating outcome of mental illness, is of particular concern to policymakers and others.

Suicide

In 2009, the suicide rate for military members serving on active duty was 18.3 per 100,000, the highest since 1980. The following year, that rate dropped to 17.0. In the general population, by comparison, the suicide rate in 2007 was 20.8 among males ages 20 to 24 and 20.7 among males ages 25 to 34.[1] From 2003 to 2010, the Department of Defense (DoD) confirmed nearly 2,000 suicides among active-duty service members, 300 of which occurred during deployment. Roughly 50 percent of suicides in 2010 occurred among military members who had deployed to overseas contingency operations. Suicide rates were higher in the Army and Marine Corps than in other branches of the military. Suicides among service members who deployed to overseas contingency operations also occur after they leave military service.

Studies of Vietnam veterans reveal that deployment to a war zone is associated with suicide in the years immediately following deployment.[2] However, information on suicides among veterans is less complete than it is for active- duty personnel, and no nationwide surveillance system exists for tracking the incidence of suicides in that population.

The Centers for Disease Control and Prevention (CDC) compiles national statistics on suicide, but veteran status and the cause of death are not always reported correctly on death certificates or summarized accurately by local health officials. CDC estimates that about 35,000 suicides occurred in the U.S. population in 2007. A separate system, the CDC's National Violent Death Reporting System—which maintains more comprehensive data on violent deaths but operates in only a limited number of states—estimates that veterans accounted for 20 percent of the suicides in those states in 2005. The CDC and Department of Veterans Affairs have ongoing initiatives to tabulate all suicides among veterans.

Statistics from VHA's suicide-prevention coordinators indicate that in fiscal year 2009 there were nearly 11,000 suicide attempts among veterans receiving care from the agency; 6.2 percent were documented as fatal. Among VHA's patients in 2007, the rate of suicide was 35 per 100,000, a rate higher than that found in the general population. However, that rate is not adjusted for the demographics of VHA's user population. Veterans who use VHA, moreover, may do so because they have more medical conditions, including mental health conditions, than other veterans or members of the general population.

As part of VHA's expansion of mental health services, the agency's suicide-prevention program is wideranging.[3] Initiatives include screening OCO veterans for selected mental health conditions; establishing suicide-prevention programs in each VHA hospital and large community-based outpatient clinic; operating a 24-hour suicide-prevention hotline staffed by VHA mental health professionals; and developing a system for flagging the records of patients at high risk of suicide.

Mental Illness

Among OCO veterans using VHA's services from October 2001 through June 2011, 21 percent were diagnosed with a depressive disorder. Other mental health conditions commonly diagnosed among OCO veterans are anxiety and drug or alcohol abuse. OCO patients with mental health conditions often have multiple conditions of this type.

Treatment for mental illness is provided at local facilities in broad consultation with VHA's Office of Mental Health Services, which has been implementing recommendations from its comprehensive five-year Mental Health Strategic Plan.

That plan, which focused on gaps in mental health care for veterans, had several goals, which included addressing the mental health needs of OCO veterans and preventing suicide. One of the steps being taken to achieve those goals is to better integrate mental health treatment and primary care. For fiscal year 2010, VHA obligated $5.2 billion for mental health programs—more than a tenth of its total spending for medical care; obligations are slated to exceed $6 billion by 2012.[4]

Available services consist of outpatient specialty programs, inpatient psychiatric care, residential and vocational rehabilitation, substance use disorder care, and various local initiatives.

VHA provided CBO with information on the use of VHA's health care services and the costs of providing those services for 73,000 OCO veterans who had a mental health diagnosis other than PTSD (and no diagnosis of TBI).

When compared with OCO veterans with no mental health diagnosis, patients with mental health disorders other than PTSD made greater use of VHA's health services in treatment year 1 as measured by inpatient hospital days (0.6 per year compared with 0.08 per year for veterans with no mental health diagnosis), annual outpatient visits (16 versus 8), and prescriptions filled (9 versus 3). When compared to OCO patients with PTSD, patients with other mental health conditions spent the same share (one-quarter) of their hospital days in psychiatric care but used less health care overall. For the first year of treatment, VHA spent $350 million on patients with other mental health diagnoses. The average cost of care during the first year of treatment ($4,300) was more than double that for OCO patients with no mental health diagnoses ($2,000) but only half the average cost of treating OCO patients with PTSD.

[1] Historically, rates of death for all causes have been lower among service members than in the general population.
[2] Institute of Medicine, *Gulf War and Health*, vol. 6, *Deployment-Related Stress and Health Outcomes* (Washington, D.C.: National Academies Press, 2007).
[3] See the Joshua Omvig Veterans Suicide Prevention Act (P.L. 110-110, 38 U.S.C. 1720F).
[4] An obligation is a commitment that creates a legal liability on the part of the government to pay for goods and services ordered or received. Such payments may be made immediately or in the future. Obligations during any year may exceed appropriations provided during that year because an agency may obligate funds that were provided in an earlier year.

CBO measured the use of services by the number of patients who used VHA's services after a diagnosis of PTSD or TBI and by the frequency of their use after those diagnoses. CBO measured VHA's services in three categories: inpatient care (in days), outpatient care (in number of clinic visits), and pharmacy services (in 30-day equivalent prescriptions filled). CBO calculated the average use by service type in each treatment year for veterans who ever used VHA's services. Patients who had PTSD, TBI, or both conditions used the VHA system much more in any given year and were more likely to use VHA's services than were patients with neither diagnosis. (This section of the analysis focuses on all health care services provided to patients in each group, regardless of whether a particular service was related to a PTSD or TBI diagnosis.) CBO found the highest average use of all health care services among patients who were treated for both PTSD and TBI. The use of services by TBI patients was roughly comparable to that of PTSD patients in the first two treatment years, but TBI patients (probably those with moderate to severe TBI) had markedly higher inpatient and outpatient use in treatment years 3 and 4. With the implementation of comprehensive screening for mild TBI in 2007, patients with moderate to severe TBI accounted for a larger share of cases in treatment years 3 and 4. Veterans with neither condition used VHA the least, with little change over the four treatment years. Use of services for most groups was highest in the first year of care.

Number of Patients Using VHA's Services

The share of veterans who continued to access care at VHA declined in the years following their initial use of its services; however, the rate of decline differed among the groups CBO analyzed. The largest decrease occurred in the group that had no diagnosis of either PTSD or TBI; less than half (42 percent) of those veterans continued to use VHA four years after initial use (see Figure 1).

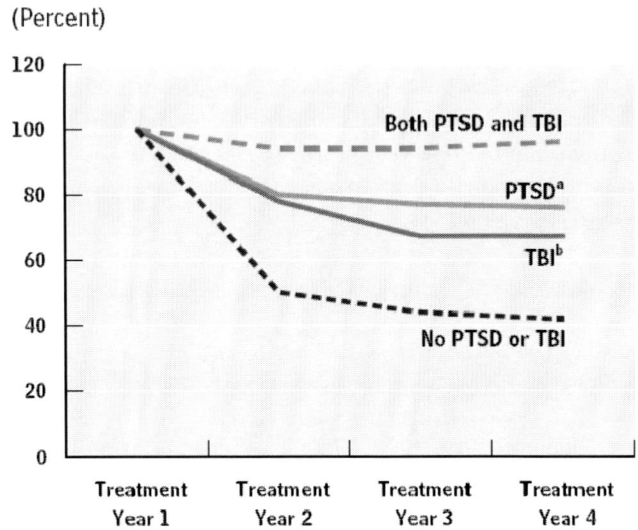

Source: Congressional Budget Office based on data from the Department of Veterans Affairs, Veterans Health Administration.

Notes: For treatment years 2 through 4, the share of patients treated by VHA represents the number of patients using VHA's services divided by the number of potential patients—those who were diagnosed with the condition in treatment year 1 and who remain in the sample (see Table D-1).

Data cover fiscal years 2004 to 2009 for up to the first four years of treatment. Data exclude about 500 patients, many with PTSD and TBI, who entered VHA at Polytrauma Rehabilitation Centers.

VHA = Veterans Health Administration; OCO = overseas contingency operations; PTSD = post-traumatic stress disorder; TBI = traumatic brain injury.

[a] Patients in the PTSD group did not have TBI, but many had other conditions.

[b] Patients in the TBI group did not have PTSD, but many had other conditions.

Figure 1. Continuation of Use of VHA's Services by OCO Veterans.

By contrast, at least two-thirds of veterans in the other three groups continued to use VHA for some of their health care four years after initial diagnosis. Those patients might have had more clinically complicated conditions that took longer to resolve. In addition, those patients' more intensive initial use of services might have predisposed them to continue pursuing care. Because of their conditions, moreover, some patients could also have had limited opportunities for employment, a common source of alternative health care options.

Frequency of Use

OCO veterans using any health care services at VHA at least once, for up to four years after diagnosis or entry into the system, were included in the calculations. Generally, OCO patients used VHA's services most intensively in the first year of treatment, after which use declined and stabilized (see Figure 2). The most notable exception was for patients with TBI (including those with both PTSD and TBI); their average use in each service category increased in treatment years 3 and 4. Patients who had neither a diagnosis of PTSD nor a diagnosis of TBI averaged many fewer inpatient days, outpatient visits, and pharmacy prescriptions than members of the other groups.[39]

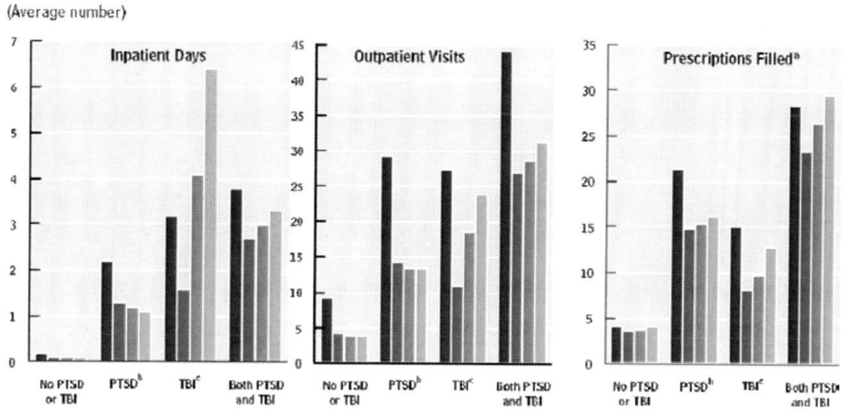

Source: Congressional Budget Office based on data from the Department of Veterans Affairs, Veterans Health Administration.

Notes: Data cover fiscal years 2004 to 2009 for up to the first four years of treatment. Data exclude about 500 patients, many with PTSD and TBI, who entered VHA at Polytrauma Rehabilitation Centers.

Average annual use is based on the number of OCO patients who were ever seen at VHA, regardless of whether they were treated in a given year.

VHA = Veterans Health Administration; OCO = overseas contingency operations; PTSD = post-traumatic stress disorder; TBI = traumatic brain injury.

[a] "Prescriptions filled" includes all pharmacy services, such as dispensing of pharmaceuticals and over-the-counter drugs (measured in 30-day equivalents), as well as related supplies.

[b] Patients in the PTSD group did not have TBI, but many had other conditions.

[c] Patients in the TBI group did not have PTSD, but many had other conditions.

Figure 2. Use of VHA's Health Care Services by OCO Patients.

Inpatient Care

Inpatient care for patients who had neither a PTSD nor a TBI diagnosis averaged less than one day in all of the years following their first visit.[40] The largest single category of inpatient care for this group in treatment year 1 was medical or surgical care (accounting for 41 percent). By contrast, the PTSD group averaged about two inpatient days in treatment year 1: 44 percent of those days were for residential rehabilitation (often treatment for mental health and substance abuse that focuses on community reintegration), and 27 percent were for psychiatric care. The TBI group averaged about three inpatient days in treatment year 1: 33 percent of those days were for rehabilitation medicine (treatment for physical impairments and disability), and 27 percent were for medical or surgical care. That distribution changed dramatically in the later years. The small number of TBI patients receiving VHA care in treatment year 4 (400 patients) were resource intensive: Inpatient hospital days for TBI patients doubled from about three in treatment year 1 to about six in treatment year 4. By treatment year 4, nursing home care, which was concentrated among fewer than 10 percent of TBI patients seeking care in that year, accounted for 82 percent of that group's inpatient days.

The final group—those with both PTSD and TBI diagnoses—averaged nearly four inpatient days in year 1. Their inpatient use was most similar to that of the PTSD group, with 39 percent of inpatient days for residential rehabilitation and 21 percent for psychiatric care.

Outpatient Care

The PTSD group's use of outpatient care in treatment year 1 was more than three times as high (29 visits) as that of OCO veterans with neither PTSD nor TBI but fell by about half (to 14 visits) in the following year and then leveled off.[41] Although the TBI group had approximately the same number of outpatient clinic visits as the PTSD group in treatment years 1 and 2, the average number of visits for the TBI group rose again in treatment years 3 and 4.

By treatment year 4, the average number of visits for the TBI group (24 visits) was close to the number in the initial year of treatment (28 visits). Again, that pattern was most likely caused by the change in screening for TBI that led to more patients with mild TBI appearing in these data in earlier treatment years than later ones. Average use of outpatient care by the group with both PTSD and TBI diagnoses decreased sharply after treatment year 1 (from 44 visits to 27 visits in treatment year 2) and then rose a little thereafter.

In the first treatment year, one-quarter of the PTSD group's outpatient visits took place in mental health clinics, and an additional 8 percent of visits were in specialty PTSD clinics. For the group with TBI, 30 percent of outpatient care was provided in the aggregated, nonspecific category of "other clinics" (which included rehabilitation clinics), and 28 percent was provided in diagnostic testing venues; less than 1 percent of their outpatient care was provided in TBI clinics.

For the group with both PTSD and TBI, 22 percent of outpatient visits in treatment year 1 occurred in mental health clinics. Data provided to CBO for this study did not include sufficient information on individual clinical encounters to report the initiation or completion of a course of therapy.

Pharmacy Services

The group with neither a PTSD nor TBI diagnosis averaged four prescriptions annually in all treatment years.[42] The other groups had considerably more pharmacy services in the first year, from four to seven times as many as the group with no PTSD or TBI diagnosis. Although pharmacy services for the other three groups—those diagnosed with PTSD, TBI, or both— decreased between treatment years 1 and 2, that decline was reversed in later years. Indeed, the group of patients with both PTSD and TBI not only had more pharmacy services, on average, in treatment year 4 than in treatment year 1 but also had the highest average number of prescriptions (30 in treatment year 4).

COSTS OF VHA'S SERVICES

Costs generally followed the same patterns as use of services. Thus, the highest average costs were for patients treated for both TBI and PTSD. Average costs for all groups of OCO patients dropped in the second year of treatment and, for most groups, stabilized or declined thereafter. A notable exception was the group of patients treated for TBI; the average costs for those patients grew substantially in treatment years 3 and 4. That apparent anomaly most likely reflects the changing composition of the TBI group during the four-year treatment period. Because the data included veterans using VHA both before and after comprehensive TBI screening was implemented, patients with mild TBI probably accounted for a larger share of cases during the first two treatment years, and patients with moderate or severe TBI represented a greater share of cases during the latter two treatment years. Because VHA did not provide data that would enable CBO to separate mild cases of TBI from moderate or severe cases, CBO's ability to examine this issue further is limited.

CBO used two different approaches to analyze VHA's costs of treating veterans with PTSD, TBI, or both. The first method captures the total costs to VHA of treating those patients but overstates costs related solely to PTSD or TBI. The second method attempts to attribute costs for services directly to a diagnosis of PTSD or TBI, which yields costs that are lower than those estimated using the first method. However, the PTSD- and TBI-specific costs can be considered only rough approximations.

In the first approach, CBO calculated the total cost of all health care provided to OCO patients diagnosed with PTSD and TBI, regardless of whether that care was directly related to those conditions. If patients were treated for a back injury or hearing loss, for example, those treatment costs were included in CBO's estimates. All costs were included because determining which care is related to a specific condition requires subjective decisions. Furthermore, patients with PTSD or TBI frequently develop other conditions that may be caused or exacerbated by the presence of PTSD or TBI and thus may be considered additional, indirect costs of PTSD and TBI.

The second approach that CBO used to compute costs was to examine only PTSD- and TBI- specific care using the diagnostic codes identified by VHA's clinicians. Determining the cost of treating a particular condition (rather than the cost of treating a patient with the condition) requires subjective decisions that attribute a medical encounter and a specific portion of the cost of that encounter to a particular condition. Computing PTSD-and TBI-specific costs, therefore, provides a rough estimate of how much VHA spends on treating those particular conditions. (See Appendix B for a description of CBO's methodology.)

Costs of All Health Care

In calculating total costs of all health care for patients with a particular diagnosis, CBO examined up to four years of data. CBO included all patients in the average cost calculations, whether those patients accessed VHA once or many times in the four years. (For an alternative method of examining average costs, see Appendix D.) Because the data are through 2009, patients that enrolled in 2007, 2008, and 2009 were not able to accumulate four years of treatment (see Appendix B).

Total Costs

During fiscal years 2004 through 2009, VHA spent $3.7 billion for the first four years of treatment on the OCO patients analyzed by CBO.[43] CBO estimates that VHA spent 60 percent of that sum ($2.2 billion) on patients with PTSD, TBI, or both. The group with neither a PTSD nor a TBI diagnosis— the largest group, with more than 350,000 patients— had the highest total costs: $860 million in treatment year 1 and about $1.5 billion in total costs from 2004 through 2009 (see Table 1). Total spending in those years for the PTSD patients was almost as high ($1.4 billion), although the PTSD group had many fewer patients.

Table 1. Total Costs for VHA's Health Care Provided to OCO Patients

Treatment Group	Total Costs (Millions of dollars)	Total Costs Attributed to PTSD- and TBI-Specific Care (Millions of dollars)	Share of Total Costs Attributed to PTSD-and TBI-Specific Care (Percent)
PTSD or TBI			
PTSD[a]	1,420	660	46
TBI[b]	130	50	38
Both PTSD and TBI	670	380	57
All PTSD and TBI	2,220	1,090	49
No PTSD or TBI	1,450	0	0
All OCO Patients	3,670	1,090	30

Source: Congressional Budget Office based on data from the Department of Veterans Affairs, Veterans Health Administration.

Notes: Data cover fiscal years 2004 to 2009 for up to the first four years of treatment. Data exclude about 500 patients, many with PTSD and TBI, who entered VHA at Polytrauma Rehabilitation Centers.

VHA converted costs provided to CBO to fiscal year 2009 dollars on the basis of annual increases in the average cost of a primary care visit from 2004 to 2009. CBO then indexed those costs to 2011 dollars using the implicit price deflator for gross domestic product.

VHA = Veterans Health Administration; OCO = overseas contingency operations; PTSD = post-traumatic stress disorder; TBI = traumatic brain injury.

[a] Patients in the PTSD group did not have TBI, but many had other conditions.

[b] Patients in the TBI group did not have PTSD, but many had other conditions.

The share of total costs devoted to inpatient care varied by treatment group but was fairly stable over the first four years of treatment for all groups except TBI patients. For most groups, the share of total costs devoted to inpatient care was less than 25 percent. For TBI patients, however, the portion of total costs assigned to inpatient care was 40 percent in treatment year 1 and 50 percent in treatment year 4. A small percentage of TBI patients were responsible for those costs: Fewer than 10 percent of TBI patients in treatment year 4 used nursing home care, but at an average cost of approximately $147,000 per nursing home patient.

Average Costs

In treatment year 1, the average costs per patient diagnosed with PTSD ($8,300), TBI ($11,700), or both ($13,800) were much higher than the average costs for those with neither PTSD nor TBI ($2,400) (see Table 2 and Figure 3 on page 20).[44] Although patients with PTSD, TBI, or both had higher average costs, those costs may not be solely attributable to those two conditions. If patients with PTSD or TBI have worse health overall (they may be more likely to have combat injuries, for example) than patients without those conditions, their costs will be higher. The group with both PTSD and TBI included patients with persistent symptoms from multiple conditions, which helps explain why their use of medical services and the costs of those services were greater than those for patients with PTSD or TBI alone.

For all groups, the average cost of all health care was highest in treatment year 1 (see Figure 3). For three of the four groups, costs largely stabilized or continued to drop in the third and fourth treatment years.

TBI patients were different. After dropping below the treatment year 1 level in years 2 and 3, costs rebounded to $11,100 in treatment year 4. That pattern can be attributed to the composition of the TBI sample in later treatment years.

As discussed earlier, the change in TBI screening implemented in 2007 means that the sample of patients analyzed here had a larger share with moderate or severe TBI in later treatment years.[45] Thus, this result does not imply that new TBI patients will tend to require higher expenditures for treatment in later years.

Costs of PTSD- and TBI-Specific Care

To provide a rough estimate of how much VHA spent on treatment specific to PTSD and TBI, CBO also presents tabulations of the costs of care that had an accompanying diagnosis code of PTSD, TBI, or both. CBO reports two types of costs for patients in the years after diagnosis: total costs and average costs for PTSD- or TBI-specific care.

The costs calculated using this method are lower than those presented earlier because they represent only a portion of health care costs for patients, not all costs.

Costs in this section should be considered a rough approximation of the costs of treating PTSD or TBI; they may be either too high or too low. When multiple diagnoses were made during an inpatient stay or outpatient visit that also included a PTSD or TBI diagnosis, VHA attributed all costs for that visit to PTSD or TBI. In addition, CBO attributed all costs for prescriptions and diagnostic tests to either PTSD or TBI for patients with those diagnoses (although VHA's clinical information systems do not associate diagnosis codes with those services).[46] That approach may overstate the costs to treat those conditions.

Conversely, patients with PTSD and TBI often have other medical problems that may be related to their PTSD or TBI and that pose indirect costs not included; in such instances, the estimates may be too low. In addition, oversights on the part of care providers or medical coders may have resulted in missing PTSD or TBI diagnosis codes, which also could produce estimates that are too low.

Total Costs

While PTSD and TBI accounted for a sizable part of total health care costs, OCO veterans with PTSD or TBI also received a considerable amount of care for other conditions, even in the first year of treatment.

VHA spent $1.1 billion for PTSD- and TBI-specific care during the 2004–2009 period for the first four years of treatment, with more than half of that amount spent on patients in their first year (see Table 1 on page 18).

For the PTSD group, PTSD-specific care averaged almost half (46 percent) of total health care costs over four years. The share was somewhat less (38 percent) for TBIspecific care for the TBI group. More than half (57 percent) of the care provided to the group with both PTSD and TBI was directly related to those specific diagnoses.

Table 2. Average Costs for All of VHA's Health Care and VHA's PTSD- and TBI-Specific Care Provided to OCO Patients (Dollars)

Treatment Group	Treatment Year 1	Treatment Year 2	Treatment Year 3	Treatment Year 4
	Average Costs per Patient			
PTSD or TBI PTSD[a]	8,300	4,200	3,900	3,800
TBIb	11,700	4,600	7,300	11,100
Both PTSD and TBI	13,800	8,400	8,800	9,800
No PTSD or TBI	2,400	1,100	1,000	1,000
	Average Costs per Patient for PTSD- and TBI-Specific Care			
PTSD	4,100	2,100	1,900	1,900
TBI	5,000	1,600	2,500	4,400
Both PTSD and TBI	8,000	4,900	5,300	5,700

Source: Congressional Budget Office based on data from the Department of Veterans Affairs, Veterans Health Administration.

Notes: Data cover fiscal years 2004 to 2009 for up to the first four years of treatment. Data exclude about 500 patients, many with PTSD and TBI, who entered VHA at Polytrauma Rehabilitation Centers.

Average annual costs are based on the number of OCO patients who were ever seen at VHA, regardless of whether they were treated in a given year.

VHA converted costs provided to CBO to fiscal year 2009 dollars on the basis of annual increases in the average cost of a primary care visit from 2004 to 2009. CBO then indexed those costs to 2011 dollars using the implicit price deflator for gross domestic product.

VHA = Veterans Health Administration; PTSD = post-traumatic stress disorder; TBI = traumatic brain injury; OCO = overseas contingency operations.

[a] Patients in the PTSD group did not have TBI, but many had other conditions.

[b] Patients in the TBI group did not have PTSD, but many had other conditions.

Average Costs

CBO's estimates of average annual costs for treating PTSD or TBI or both in patients with those diagnoses can be regarded only as rough estimates because of the broad classification of treatments attributable to PTSD or TBI. Following the initial year of treatment for patients with PTSD, which cost $4,100 per patient for PTSD-specific care, those costs fell by about half (see Table 2).

Average costs of treating veterans with both PTSD- and TBI-specific care in year 1 ($8,000 per patient) were almost double those for veterans with PTSD alone, and $3,000 higher than the average costs of treating patients with TBI alone.

Between treatment year 1 and treatment year 4, the average costs of care for PTSD and combined PTSD and TBI declined by 54 percent and 29 percent, respectively, but the average costs of TBI care decreased by only 12 percent during that period.

As noted above, the pattern of costs for veterans with TBI is distorted by the change in screening during the sample period.

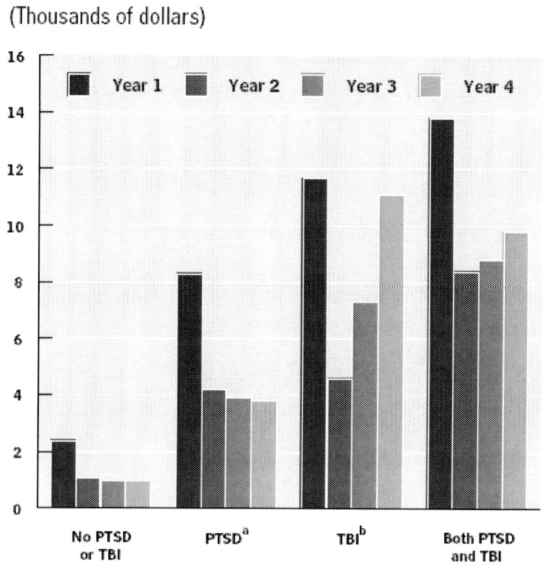

Source: Congressional Budget Office based on data from the Department of Veterans Affairs, Veterans Health Administration.

Notes: Data cover fiscal years 2004 to 2009 for up to the first four years of treatment. Data exclude about 500 patients, many with PTSD and TBI, who entered VHA at Polytrauma Rehabilitation Centers.

Average annual costs are based on the number of OCO patients who were ever seen at VHA, regardless of whether they were treated in a given year.

VHA converted costs provided to CBO to fiscal year 2009 dollars on the basis of annual increases in the average cost of a primary care visit from 2004 to 2009. CBO then indexed those costs to 2011 dollars using the implicit price deflator for gross domestic product.

VHA = Veterans Health Administration; OCO = overseas contingency operations; PTSD = post-traumatic stress disorder; TBI = traumatic brain injury.

[a] Patients in the PTSD group did not have TBI, but many had other conditions.

[b] Patients in the TBI group did not have PTSD, but many had other conditions.

Figure 3. Average Costs for All of VHA's Health Care Provided to OCO Patients.

Other Studies of the Costs of Treating PTSD and TBI

CBO reviewed other studies on the costs of treating people with PTSD and TBI. CBO focused on studies examining those conditions in the OCO population, in part because costs experienced by the civilian population are unlikely to be comparable to those for the military population.[47] While studies of the costs to treat OCO veterans have been limited, more research is becoming available. CBO reviewed two studies of VHA costs, neither of which attempted to examine the costs of care related specifically to PTSD or TBI.

One study compared the costs of treating OCO veterans with PTSD or TBI with the costs of treating OCO veterans without those conditions.[48] In fiscal year 2008, the average cost for patients with PTSD alone was between $6,000 and $8,000 (expressed in 2011 dollars), and the average cost for patients with TBI totaled about $5,000. (TBI cases in that study were identified through VHA's screening and therefore were more likely to have been mild and less expensive to treat.) The corresponding cost for patients with both PTSD and TBI was $10,300. For veterans with neither condition, the average cost was $2,500, very similar to CBO's estimate for treatment year 1. Compared with CBO's estimates, most costs reported in the study for fiscal year 2008 are lower, but CBO's data contained a different mix of cases that included more severe ones.

A second study examined the average costs in fiscal year 2009 for VHA to treat OCO patients who had used any outpatient services in that year. The cost estimates, therefore, were for patients who first sought care in 2009, as well as those who had been treated for several years. The authors found that the median annual cost per patient with PTSD was $2,800 (expressed in 2011 dollars); the mean was $5,300. For patients with TBI, the median cost was $3,400, and the mean was $7,300. For veterans with both PTSD and TBI, the median cost was $7,300, and the mean was $12,300.[49] Those average values for fiscal year 2009 are all lower than CBO's estimates of all health care costs for such patients for the first treatment year.

Another study, by the RAND Corporation, examined costs of treating service members who deployed to overseas contingency operations, but its focus on societal costs makes it dissimilar to CBO's analysis of VHA's costs.[50]

POLYTRAUMA PATIENTS

Polytrauma patients at VHA are those with multiple severe injuries. Patients categorized as polytrauma for purposes of this analysis first enrolled in the VHA system as inpatients at one of the Polytrauma Rehabilitation Centers; about 500 OCO veterans were identified as polytrauma patients. Some patients with multiple traumas were included in other groups in CBO's analysis, however, because their first encounters with VHA were not at a Polytrauma Rehabilitation Center, but rather at some other facility.

After initial entry into the polytrauma system, those patients continued to access VHA's health care system. In any given treatment year, at least 95 percent used VHA and had some PTSD- and TBI-specific care. Like patients in the other groups, polytrauma patients used significantly more resources in treatment year 1 than in later years (see Table 3). The average hospital stay in treatment year 1 was close to two months, with 73 percent of that care delivered in rehabilitation medicine. In subsequent years, the average annual length of an inpatient stay declined dramatically. Outpatient clinic visits for polytrauma patients were close to half the initial number by treatment year 4. Pharmacy use declined 36 percent in treatment year 2, but as with other groups analyzed in this study, increased thereafter.

The pattern of use was reflected in the costs of treatment. The average cost of all health care per polytrauma patient in treatment year 1 was $136,000, or nearly 10 times the average cost for the group with both PTSD and TBI. Average annual health care costs dropped to about 30 percent of their first-year amount in treatment year 2 and to about 20 percent of that amount by year 4. PTSD- and TBI-specific care accounted for 60 percent ($55 million) of total health care costs for polytrauma patients during the 2004–2009 period, a percentage similar to that for the group with both PTSD and TBI.[51] In total, health care costs for the roughly 500 polytrauma patients treated between 2004 and 2009 exceeded $91 million.

Table 3. Use and Costs of VHA's Health Care Provided to OCO Polytrauma Patients

	Treatment Year 1	Treatment Year 2	Treatment Year 3	Treatment Year 4
	Average Use per Patient			
Inpatient Days	56	17	8	11
Outpatient Visits	77	66	60	43
Prescriptions Filled[a]	45	29	31	33
	Average Costs per Patient (Dollars)			
Health Care	136,000	42,000	27,000	28,000

Source: Congressional Budget Office based on data from the Department of Veterans Affairs, Veterans Health Administration. Notes: Data cover fiscal years 2004 to 2009 for up to the first four years of treatment.

Average annual use and costs are based on the number of OCO patients who were ever seen at VHA, regardless of whether they were treated in a given year.

VHA converted costs provided to CBO to fiscal year 2009 dollars on the basis of annual increases in the average cost of a primary care visit from 2004 to 2009. CBO then indexed those costs to 2011 dollars using the implicit price deflator for gross domestic product.

VHA = Veterans Health Administration; OCO = overseas contingency operations.

[a] "Prescriptions filled" includes all pharmacy services, such as the dispensing of pharmaceuticals and over-the-counter drugs (measured in 30-day equivalents), as well as related supplies.

APPENDIX A: BACKGROUND ON PTSD AND TBI

Post-traumatic stress disorder (PTSD) is an anxiety disorder induced by exposure to a traumatic event. Although the psychological effects of combat have long been recognized (in previous wars, the symptoms now associated with PTSD were known as "shell shock" or "battle fatigue"), the American Psychiatric Association did not codify PTSD as a separate mental disorder until 1980. Traumatic brain injuries (TBIs) are defined as a blow, jolt, or penetrating injury to the head that interrupts the functioning of the brain, at least momentarily. Medical intervention varies considerably. During military combat operations, some mild TBIs may go untreated when there are no physical head wounds or neurological signs of impairment. Medical personnel may not detect injury, especially when more obvious, life-threatening injuries require attention, and service members may not seek care for a TBI if the injury does not appear acute. Moderate and severe TBIs, however, are generally apparent clinically through changes in consciousness or neurological impairment.

Criteria for a PTSD Diagnosis

According to current diagnostic criteria for PTSD, a person must experience a traumatic event—involving death or serious injury, or a threat to the physical integrity of self or others—and react to the trauma with intense horror, fear, or helplessness.[1] Sometime after that trauma, the person must also develop symptoms that cause clinically significant distress or impairment lasting for more than one month. Those symptoms must be from each of the following three symptom clusters:

- Reexperiencing the traumatic event, such as having recurring and distressing recollections or nightmares;
- Avoidance of stimuli associated with the trauma, such as thoughts, feelings, and conversations, along with diminished responsiveness and loss of interest in activities; and
- Hyperarousal, such as irritability, anger, hyper-vigilance, insomnia, or difficulty with concentration.

For example, a person who experienced nightmares about the trauma and had lost interest in daily activities but had no symptoms of hyperarousal would not have PTSD, according to those diagnostic criteria.

There are various forms of PTSD. Acute PTSD occurs when the duration of symptoms is between one and three months. Patients with symptoms extending for more than three months are considered to have chronic PTSD. Delayed-onset PTSD occurs when symptoms begin at least six months after the trauma.

Course of PTSD

Among people who develop PTSD, the symptoms and their intensity may differ over the course of the disorder.[2] Some people recover without medical intervention; others experience chronic symptoms persisting for years, even decades; and still others have sporadic symptoms. For most people who develop PTSD, symptoms appear soon after the trauma, although the time between exposure and symptoms sufficient for a clinical diagnosis of PTSD varies.

Studies of Vietnam veterans who developed PTSD have found that, for most veterans, the onset of PTSD occurred during the first few years following combat trauma, with the number of symptoms increasing rapidly during that period. A study by Schnurr reported that more than 60 percent of Vietnam veterans who developed PTSD did so less than two years after entry into the combat theater; fewer than 10 percent experienced an onset of PTSD more than six years after entering the combat theater.

Researchers have found that a substantial portion of PTSD patients develop chronic PTSD. Two studies— one by Breslau and one by Kessler and others—indicate that, for 20 percent to 40 percent of PTSD cases, symptoms abate within one year. According to Kessler and others, as well as Conner and Butterfield, symptoms do not improve substantially in more than one-third of PTSD cases even after several years. (Because the populations, treatment, and timing of treatment in those studies differ from those in CBO's analysis, the rates of remission reported in the studies may not be applicable to more recent combat veterans.)

Risk and protective factors for experiencing PTSD and for subsequent recovery include demographic characteristics, socioeconomic status, psychiatric history, and social support. Among Vietnam veterans, women were more likely than men to develop PTSD. Research also shows that lower educational attainment, lower income, and minority status place individuals at greater risk.[3] The presence of social networks and social support after a stressor serves to protect against PTSD, particularly for combat veterans. Finally, more frequent and intense exposure to combat is strongly associated with the development of PTSD.

Clinical Definition of TBI

The Centers for Disease Control and Prevention defines TBI as an injury to the head arising from blunt or penetrating trauma or from acceleration-deceleration forces that result in one or more of the following:

- decreased level of consciousness;
- amnesia regarding the event itself or events preceding or following the injury;
- skull fracture;
- a neurological or neuropsychological abnormality such as disorientation, agitation, or confusion; or
- an intracranial lesion such as a traumatic intracranial hematoma, cerebral contusion, or penetrating injury.[4]

Neurologists classify the severity of the TBI at the time of the injury as mild, moderate, or severe. Mild TBIs account for the vast majority of such injuries. Definitions of mild TBI, also known as a concussion, vary within the neurology community, but a generally accepted definition from the American Congress of Rehabilitation Medicine specifies at least one of the following symptoms after a blow to the head:

- Loss of consciousness for no more than 30 minutes;
- Loss of memory, lasting no longer than 24 hours, of events immediately before (retrograde amnesia) or after (posttraumatic amnesia) the injury;
- Any alteration in mental state (being dazed, disoriented, or confused, for example) at the time of the injury; or
- A score of 13 to 15 on a Glasgow coma scale (an assessment of neurological functioning).[5]

Injuries above any of those thresholds are moderate to severe TBIs. The continuation of multiple symptoms may be labeled as postconcussional disorder or post-concussive syndrome (PCS); however, those terms are problematic because there is no single clinically validated definition of the condition.[6] Short- or long-term impairment may affect memory, reasoning and problem solving, language, speech, motor skills, physical functions, and psychosocial behavior.

Course of TBI

Although the effects of, and recovery from, TBI differ among individuals, impairment tends to be greater for those with moderate or severe TBIs than for those with mild TBIs. Moderate and severe TBIs are usually associated with damage to the brain that can be detected when imaged.[7] For people with moderate or severe TBI, injuries to the brain—swelling of brain tissue, insufficient blood flow, and pressure within the skull, for example—may require surgery or medication. Recovery from moderate or severe TBI ranges from full rehabilitation to significant disability. Survivors of moderate or severe TBI may suffer lasting consequences such as seizures, nerve damage, behavioral abnormalities, and cognitive and language difficulties.

Research findings on the course of recovery after mild TBI vary widely, partly because of the difficulty in making causal associations between the initial injury and physical or cognitive problems following the injury.[8] Frequently reported problems following a mild TBI include headache, fatigue, dizziness, depression, and difficulties with memory and concentration. However, many problems associated with mild TBIs are nonspecific or common to many conditions and widely experienced by the general population. Consequently, there is no objective way of determining whether ongoing problems are caused by an earlier mild TBI or arise from other conditions.

Most people with mild TBI report one or more symptoms or problems immediately after the injury; however, medical evidence suggests that recovery typically occurs within a matter of weeks or months, with improvement most pronounced in the first months.[9] In addition, some studies indicate that between 5 percent and 20 percent of people who experience a mild TBI remain symptomatic after 12 months, although some researchers have reported rates that exceed 20 percent, and others have argued that rates are at the lower end of the range at most.[10] Generally, studies report that a small subset of patients experience one or more symptoms or limitations for years after the injury. Repeated incidents of mild TBI (as may occur from wartime explosions or in contact sports such as football or hockey) may lead to more significant longterm health problems.

Several studies have attempted to identify preinjury and postinjury factors that may alter the course of recovery from mild TBI.[11] Researchers have found that the severity and duration of symptoms can be reduced by providing reassurance to patients and by providing education to patients on both the course of TBI and expected recovery from the condition. Few other factors have consistently been shown to facilitate recovery from mild, symptomatic TBI.

APPENDIX B: DATA AND METHODS

The Veterans Health Administration (VHA) provided the Congressional Budget Office (CBO) with information on the frequency and costs of various health care services for veterans of overseas contingency operations (OCO) for fiscal years 2004 through 2009. VHA identified patients using a roster of OCO veterans that was derived from the Department of Defense's (DoD's) list of separated service members eligible for VHA benefits. The roster is based on a combination of pay and operational records and contains data fields describing both general demographic characteristics and military service information such as branch, rank, and deployment dates.

VHA data included virtually all OCO veterans seen at VHA during fiscal years 2004 to 2009; fewer than 1 percent of patients were deleted from the data set because their information was incomplete. VHA provided the data to CBO in groups organized by sex, age interval, year of treatment, clinical service use, and clinical diagnoses. The diagnosis groups were defined to be mutually exclusive, so that no patient was included in more than one diagnosis group during the first year of treatment at VHA; once classified, patients remained in the same group for the entire sample period. A patient was identified as having post-traumatic stress disorder (PTSD) or a traumatic brain injury (TBI) if he or she had at least one medical encounter with VHA in which PTSD or TBI was listed as a primary or secondary diagnosis. The identification of PTSD and TBI was broad, in that not all patients with those diagnoses sustained those conditions while deployed and, even among those who did sustain the conditions while deployed, the conditions were not necessarily related to combat. Patients who did not receive a diagnosis of PTSD or TBI were also followed from their first visit to VHA. From the time of the initial clinic visit or inpatient stay, all patients were followed in 12-month increments. Service use and costs were aggregated into totals by year of treatment.

CBO subsequently combined all patients into four mutually exclusive cohorts: no documented diagnosis of PTSD or TBI, a diagnosis of PTSD and not TBI, a diagnosis of TBI and not PTSD, or diagnoses of both PTSD and TBI.[1] Polytrauma patients were analyzed separately as a fifth group because their usage was greater and their costs substantially higher than those of other OCO patients. Small cohort size was an issue in later treatment years: CBO restricted its analysis to the first four years of treatment for each entry group. As overseas contingency operations have continued, increasing numbers of service members have deployed and separated from the military and become eligible for VHA care; therefore, many patients in CBO's analysis entered the VHA system in the last two years of the sample period (2008 and 2009), and data accrued for them only for treatment years 1 or 2 (see Figure B-1). Consequently, each group had fewer patients in treatment year 4 than in treatment year 1. Because CBO did not have data at the patient level, only group totals and weighted averages were calculated. The lack of patient-level data made it impossible to separate groups by the year in which patients first used VHA's services, preventing CBO from following groups of patients during the specific fiscal years in which they were treated.

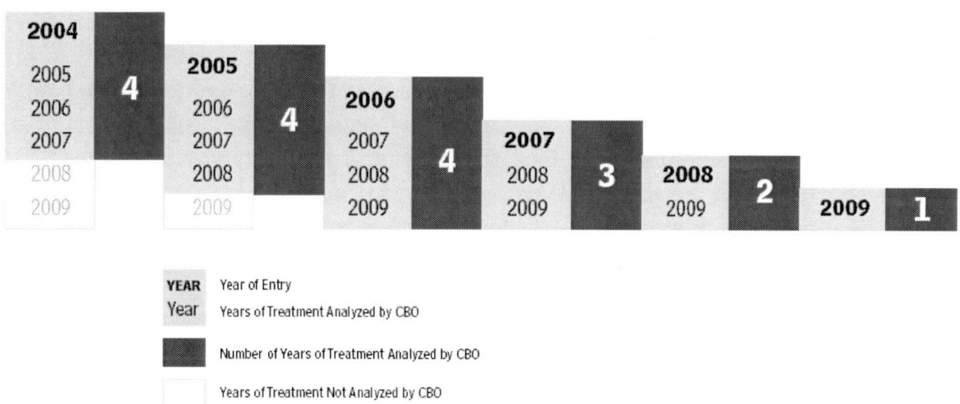

Source: Congressional Budget Office.
Notes: VHA = Veterans Health Administration; OCO = overseas contingency operations.

Figure B-1. Years of Potential Use of VIA's Services, by OCO Patient's Year of Entry.

VHA extracted data on patients' use of services mainly from its National Patient Care Database, which includes information on patients from all of its clinical information systems. Information on the use of various medical services was available for 16 detailed categories, not all of which were well populated. To provide a general overview, CBO classified the use of services as inpatient, outpatient, or outpatient pharmacy. Use was measured in days of inpatient hospital care and outpatient clinic visits. A veteran may have had several outpatient visits on a single day, each tallied separately. Pharmacy services were measured as the number of 30-day equivalent prescriptions filled.

The primary source of the cost data provided to CBO was the cost-accounting system of VHA's Decision Support Service (DSS); a second source, the Fee Basis database, included the cost of outside care paid for by VHA. VHA combined those separate sources of cost data, which captured most of the costs of services covered by VHA, into unified data for CBO. Costs reflected medical center-specific expenditures. Approximately 8 percent of total costs were not included, such as those for capital, depreciation, the central office of the Department of Veterans Affairs (VA), and some national programs. Because of those exclusions, the data used by CBO were slightly different from the DSS data available to most VHA researchers; therefore, other researchers may not be able to reproduce the same results precisely.

The DSS system takes clinical and financial information from other VHA databases and uses algorithms that merge data and allocate costs across functional units. Cost estimates of individual health care encounters are also produced. Those costs include both direct and indirect (overhead) components. Because the accuracy of those costs depends on the quality of the feeder databases, DSS data are subject to auditing at regular intervals. DSS data are longitudinal and retrospective. VHA uses DSS information extensively, including for the purpose of financial allocation, and considers the data to be highly reliable.

DSS computations to derive patient-level costs require several steps. First, cost data from VHA's core financial and payroll systems are fed into DSS. Those cost data reflect VHA's actual outlays for salaries, supplies, and contract services, as well as imputed costs for depreciation. At that level, expenditures are differentiated by type of expense (labor category or supplies and equipment) and by administrative service (nursing or laboratory tests). Next, DSS assigns costs to functional cost centers that involve either the direct provision of health care or indirect support for health care. Cost centers that provide care directly include primary care clinics and psychiatric wards, whereas cost centers that provide indirect support for health care include information technology support and security. Using a standardized methodology, those indirect costs are then allocated to departments providing care directly within each facility. After all costs have been assigned by function, unit costs for intermediate products are constructed. Intermediate products are goods and services used in providing care, such as blood draws, laboratory tests, or doctors' time during primary care visits. Finally, all intermediate products and their prices are assigned to individual patients to estimate the cost of health care encounters.[2]

CBO categorized cost data as inpatient and outpatient, with outpatient pharmacy costs included in the outpatient category. VHA converted the costs provided to CBO to fiscal year 2009 dollars on the basis of annual increases in the average cost of a primary care visit between fiscal years 2004 and 2009. CBO then indexed those costs to 2011 dollars using the implicit price deflator for gross domestic product.

Using those data, CBO calculated average costs per patient with PTSD or TBI, or both, of health care services for each treatment year by dividing costs in that year (the numerator) by the number of patients who had ever been diagnosed for PTSD or TBI and remained in the sample that year (the denominator). Average costs for those without PTSD or TBI were calculated using a similar method. Patients who used care from VHA for only a single year or a single time were included in the denominator for all subsequent years, even years for which they had no costs. In other words, CBO counted the entire population of veterans diagnosed with PTSD or TBI regardless of whether they continued to use VHA's services after their first visit. That approach shows VHA's average cost per patient to treat the entire population of veterans in each diagnosis group (those diagnosed with PTSD, TBI, both, or neither).

In calculating the average costs of PTSD- and TBIspecific care, CBO used a similar methodology. VHA provided two additional cost categories: "all PTSD care" and "all TBI care," which were used as the numerator. The tallies of those categories should be viewed as rough approximations of the costs of treating PTSD and TBI. VHA assigned all costs associated with a medical encounter (for example, an inpatient stay or outpatient visit) as "PTSD care" or "TBI care" whenever there was a primary or secondary diagnosis of either condition. For the group with both PTSD and TBI, if an encounter had both diagnosis codes, all the costs for that encounter were counted in both categories—that is, they were assigned to the costs of "PTSD care" and also to those of "TBI care"—so estimates of dollars spent for the treatment of PTSD and TBI are not mutually exclusive. For all groups, the total cost of an entire visit was attributed to PTSD or TBI (or both) even if there were several other diagnoses. CBO used VHA's "all PTSD care" and "all TBI care" cost categories and, in addition, attributed the costs of diagnostic tests and pharmacy use, to which VHA does not assign diagnosis codes, to PTSD or TBI care, according to the group to which patients had been assigned. Inclusion of diagnostic tests and pharmacy services increased the costs for the subtotals for "all PTSD care" and "all TBI care" by between 20 percent and 35 percent.

Appendix C: Interpreting Published Estimates of the Prevalence of PTSD and TBI

Prevalence estimates for post-traumatic stress disorder (PTSD) and traumatic brain injury (TBI) vary substantially. Changes in diagnostic criteria over time, as well as differences in the populations studied, diagnostic tools used to identify cases, and the methodologies employed all contribute to that variation.

PTSD Prevalence among Current Service Members Who Deployed to Overseas Contingency Operations and Veterans of Those Operations

PTSD was first included in the American Psychiatric Association's *Diagnosis and Statistical Manual of Mental Disorders* in 1980; for a diagnosis of PTSD, a person must have experienced a traumatic event and certain symptoms related to that trauma. A number of studies have addressed PTSD in service members or veterans. Estimates of the proportion of service members with PTSD generally range between 5 percent and 25 percent, depending on the study's methodology and the population sampled.[1]

Some observers have looked to the prevalence of PTSD among veterans of the Vietnam War. Widely quoted is the National Vietnam Veterans Readjustment Study (NVVRS), an extensive survey and analysis of mental health problems among Vietnam War veterans. Researchers using those data estimated that 15 percent of male Vietnam-theater veterans had combat-related PTSD at the time of the survey (1988), and 31 percent had experienced combat-related PTSD at some point in their lives prior to the survey.[2] A more recent reanalysis of a subsample of the NVVRS data found lower prevalence rates of 9 percent and lifetime prevalence of 19 percent as of 1988. The decrease in prevalence rates in the second analysis was largely attributed to a change in the methodology used to identify a case of PTSD.[3] While prevalence rates among Vietnam War veterans are important for estimating the resources that group might require for future treatment, those rates are not good indicators of the likely prevalence rates for military members who have served in the Iraq and Afghanistan conflicts. Previous research shows that various factors—demographics, educational attainment, social support, combat intensity and injuries, and past psychiatric history, among others—affect whether service members will develop PTSD, and Vietnam veterans differ from veterans recently discharged from the military in some of those respects.[4]

Several recent studies have estimated the prevalence of PTSD among those who deployed to overseas contingency operations in Iraq and Afghanistan. Many have relied on the commonly used 17-item PTSD Checklist (PCL), in which veterans report their own symptoms, to screen for PTSD; relatively few of those studies surveyed members of all four military services or included reserve and National Guard as well as active-duty personnel.[5] A 2008 RAND study based on a telephone survey of 1,965 service members and veterans who had returned from overseas contingency operations found that 14 percent screened positive for PTSD. Within that group, higher rates were observed among Army soldiers and National Guard and reserve personnel than among other groups; higher rates were observed for those with longer deployments; and higher rates were observed for those seriously injured during their deployment.[6] A separate study by Smith and others reported new cases of PTSD in as few as 1 percent to 4 percent of deployed service members in the Air Force who did not experience combat exposure, but up to 9 percent for Army soldiers who had experienced certain combat-related traumas or exposures.[7] Other studies have estimated the prevalence of PTSD from data on service members' responses to the Department of Defense's (DoD's) screening test for that condition.[8] Some estimates based on that test were on the higher end of the spectrum. For example, a study by Milliken and others found that between 6 percent and 12 percent of active Army personnel and between 6 percent and 13 percent of Army reservists screened positive for PTSD immediately upon returning from deployment to the Iraq war. The same study showed that assessments conducted three to six months after deployment yielded positive screening rates between 9 percent and 17 percent for active soldiers and between 14 percent and 25 percent for reserve soldiers.[9]

Issues in Reporting PTSD Prevalence Rates

There are two main problems in applying the published rates of PTSD to the entire population of OCO veterans. First, the studies relied on screening tools to establish a case of PTSD, and those instruments may not produce accurate estimates of the prevalence of the underlying condition. Second, the samples used in the studies were seldom representative of all personnel who deployed.

Screening Tools to Estimate PTSD Prevalence Rates

Although studies usually estimate rates of possible PTSD using a screening questionnaire, those tools do not replace a clinician-determined diagnosis. Screening questionnaires are not comprehensive and do not determine whether all relevant criteria for a diagnosis have been met.[10] Also, different researchers may use more or less stringent criteria to estimate the number of PTSD cases, which would result in dissimilar estimates even if the researchers used the same sample of service members and the identical screening tool.[11]

Finally, because screening tools are imperfect, they generate false positives and false negatives; the resulting prevalence estimates, therefore, may diverge from the true prevalence rates. For conditions in which the underlying prevalence in the population is relatively low, a screen may be more likely to overestimate the number of cases, particularly when used as a clinical tool designed to capture as many potential cases as possible.[12]

Subsamples of the OCO Population

Most of the published studies on PTSD have examined a subsample of service members who have deployed to overseas contingency operations, often combat troops in the Army or Marine Corps, and excluded the more numerous support personnel (such as truck drivers or supply handlers) or personnel from the Navy and Air Force. Although those results may be important for estimating the prevalence of PTSD in the highest-risk units, they cannot be directly applied to the entire deployed force. Other military occupations and service branches are likely to see lower levels of combat when deployed and consequently to experience lower levels of PTSD than the Army and Marine ground combat forces that have deployed, all else being equal. Even studies that attempt to survey the entire deployed force may not be representative because some service members may be more likely than others to respond to a survey. Furthermore, service members may not respond truthfully if they are concerned that reporting could result in stigma and possibly jeopardize their careers or delay their return home.[13] In addition, methodological attempts to mitigate effects of unrepresentative samples may not be wholly successful. Because of those factors, the samples analyzed may either understate or overstate the prevalence of PTSD among service members who deployed to overseas contingency operations.

TBI Prevalence among Current Service Members Who Deployed to Overseas Contingency Operations and Veterans of Those Operations

Measuring TBI in the OCO population also presents challenges. TBI results from an injury to the head, and the symptoms that follow the injury vary substantially. Research on the prevalence of TBI has been limited by inconsistent case definitions for TBI and the absence of ongoing population surveillance systems before the 1990s. Even now, the number of TBIs attributable to service in overseas contingency operations is difficult to measure. Many cases of TBI may never be recorded because medical attention may not have seemed necessary at the time of injury and because the Veterans Health Administration and the Department of Defense did not institute their population-based screening programs until 2007 and 2008, respectively.

Although investigation of the prevalence of TBI has not been as extensive as that for PTSD, some researchers have estimated the number of OCO service members who screen positive for TBI or continue to have symptoms of TBI. Researchers generally estimate that the proportion of service members deployed to overseas contingency operations who experienced a TBI (including those who were no longer symptomatic) is between 15 percent and 23 percent, depending on the study's methodology and sample; their estimates of the portion of service members who continue to experience symptoms over the longer term (that is, who continue to have symptomatic TBI) range from 4 percent to 9 percent.

A study by Hoge and others found that 15 percent of soldiers in two Army infantry brigades returning from deployment to Iraq screened positive for experiencing a mild TBI.[14] A 2008 RAND study that was based on a telephone survey of OCO service members and veterans reported a probable TBI prevalence of almost 20 percent.[15] A paper by Terrio and others estimated that 23 percent of soldiers in an Army brigade combat team returning from a one-year deployment to Iraq had experienced a TBI while deployed.[16] That paper also examined the frequency of continued medical complaints that may be attributed to TBI, including headache, irritability, dizziness, balance problems, and memory difficulties. The authors found that 9 percent of personnel within the brigade reported at least one ongoing symptom potentially related to TBI, and 4 percent reported a minimum of two ongoing symptoms at the time of the screening, a few days after returning home from deployment. By comparison, VHA researchers have found that 7 percent of OCO veterans who are screened receive a diagnosis of symptomatic TBI.[17] In part because there are no validated clinical criteria for symptomatic TBI, estimates from these studies are not comparable.

Issues in Reporting TBI Prevalence Rates

The rates of TBI reported in those published studies should not be interpreted as the prevalence for the whole population of service members deployed in support of the conflicts in Iraq and Afghanistan. Estimates of TBI in those studies are problematic for several reasons: Studies use different sets of diagnosis codes to approximate the number of TBI cases; they rely on screening instruments for TBI rather than clinical diagnoses at or near the time of injury; and they use samples that are not representative of the entire deployed force. Furthermore, even if the prevalence of TBI could be precisely determined, the extent of impairment and consequent need for continuing medical care are unknown.

Diagnosis Codes to Estimate TBI Prevalence Rates

Studies that provide estimates of TBI frequency based on diagnosis codes are problematic. For one thing, not everyone with a TBI will seek treatment and receive a diagnosis, which leads to underestimates. For another, there is no single diagnosis code to identify TBIs. The codes identify several types of injuries to the head, distinguished by the section of the head injured rather than by the severity of injury to the brain itself. Researchers have employed different collections of codes to estimate the number of TBIs.

Screening Tools to Estimate TBI Prevalence Rates

Studies have generally relied on screening tools or questions that are based on the Brief Traumatic Brain Injury Screen (BTBIS) to identify possible TBIs.[18] The BTBIS does not replace a clinician-determined diagnosis at the time of injury. Indeed, the accuracy of the BTBIS is not known because it has not been psychometrically validated against clinicians' diagnoses at or near the time of injury.

When the BTBIS is compared with a structured clinical interview that may occur several months after the injury, VHA researchers have found that the screen correctly identifies the vast majority of OCO veterans who remain symptomatic but also falsely identifies a large number of people.[19] Because the screen was designed as a clinical tool to identify as many cases of TBI as possible, studies relying on that tool are likely to overestimate, perhaps significantly, the prevalence of both TBI and TBI with persistent symptoms. Also, the timing of the screening may result in substantially different responses in the same population.[20]

Sample Selection

Sample selection is also problematic when estimating the prevalence of TBI, much as it is for PTSD. Studies have tended to focus on combat troops returning to their units. Even in the few studies that did survey active-duty personnel from all four branches of service, not just Army soldiers, certain groups of service members were either undersampled or oversampled.

Although combat troops are much more likely to experience a TBI (and thereby inflate estimates of TBI prevalence), a sample of soldiers who return to their units does not include severely injured service members who have been medically evacuated from the combat theater; excluding medical evacuees from the sample underestimates the prevalence of TBI.

Extent of Impairment

Finally, even if the number of TBIs sustained in combat theater could be accurately determined, an important issue remains in understanding the impact of TBI on the health care needs of the OCO population: The degree of impairment is unknown. Even a clinical diagnosis at or shortly after a TBI occurs indicates only that an injury was sustained; it does not reveal the persistence or intensity of symptoms at the time of the diagnosis. Indeed, the literature indicates that the vast majority of individuals who experience a mild TBI recover spontaneously over a period of a few weeks or months. In addition, for some who remain symptomatic, many of the neurological and physiological indicators and limitations arising from TBI (headaches, memory difficulties, sleep problems) are not specific to the injury and may be caused by either the TBI or other conditions, complicating clinical assessment of TBI.[21] Studies that report rates of symptomatic TBI show substantially lower rates than studies that measure the number of service members who sustained a TBI during deployment to a combat theater.

APPENDIX D: VHA'S AVERAGE ANNUAL COSTS FOR OCO VETERANS WHO CONTINUE TO SEEK CARE

In this study, the Congressional Budget Office (CBO) calculated average costs per patient of health care services for each treatment year by dividing costs in that year (the numerator) by the number of patients who ever used VHA's services and remained in the sample that year (the denominator). (For the denominator for each treatment year, see the number of potential patients in Table D-1.)

That method yields costs for specific groups of new OCO veterans, including some who used VHA only once and others who used VHA more frequently or even continually. Those results are presented in the main text of this study.

An alternative way to calculate average costs in a treatment year is to include in the denominator only those patients who continued to receive health care in each subsequent year. (For the denominator for each treatment year using that method, see the number of patients using VHA in Table D-1.) That method will produce higher annual average costs per patient, because the total cost for treating patients each year is divided by the number of patients who used services in that year (consequently, the denominator is smaller). In this appendix, CBO presents average costs using the second method.

The first approach provides the cost for treating a given group of veterans; the second approach provides the cost for treating a group of veterans who are continually seeking care.

Table D-1. Sample Sizes

Treatment Group	Patients Using VHA	Potential Patients in Group	Share of Patients Using VHA (Percent)
		Treatment Year 1	
PTSD or TBI			
PTSD[a]	103,500	103,500	100
TBI[b]	8,700	8,700	100
Both PTSD and TBI	26,600	26,600	100
No PTSD or TBI	358,000	358,000	100
		Treatment Year 2	
PTSD or TBI			
PTSD[a]	55,600	69,100	80
TBI[b]	2,800	3,600	78
Both PTSD and TBI	17,500	18,600	94
No PTSD or TBI	124,100	248,800	50
		Treatment Year 3	
PTSD or TBI			
PTSD[a]	33,600	43,800	77
TBI[b]	800	1,200	67
Both PTSD and TBI	10,000	10,600	94
No PTSD or TBI	77,400	177,800	44
		Treatment Year 4	
PTSD or TBI			
PTSD[a]	18,600	24,600	76
TBI[b]	400	600	67
Both PTSD and TBI	5,300	5,500	96
No PTSD or TBI	48,600	115,300	42

Source: Congressional Budget Office based on data from the Department of Veterans Affairs, Veterans Health Administration.

Notes: Data cover fiscal years 2004 to 2009 for up to the first four years of treatment. Data exclude 500 patients, many with PTSD and TBI, who entered VHA at Polytrauma Rehabilitation Centers.

VHA = Veterans Health Administration; PTSD = post-traumatic stress disorder; TBI = traumatic brain injury.

[a] Patients in the PTSD group did not have TBI, but many had other conditions.

[b] Patients in the TBI group did not have PTSD, but many had other conditions.

After the first year of treatment, average annual costs for patients using VHA were higher than for potential patients, because some of the potential patients had no VHA costs associated with them (see Table D-2).

Differences in average costs for the two samples were most pronounced for patients who had neither PTSD nor TBI. For that category of patients, the average cost of treatment in year 4 for patients using VHA ($2,300) was more than twice the cost for potential patients ($1,000, shown in Table 2 on page 19).

Because so many veterans with PTSD and with both PTSD and TBI continued to use VHA care, differences in average cost between the two samples were much smaller for veterans diagnosed with those conditions.

By treatment year 4, the average cost for patients using VHA with PTSD ($5,100) was 34 percent more than for potential patients with PTSD ($3,800). For veterans with both PTSD and TBI, the average annual cost for patients using VHA was only $400 more than the cost for potential patients.

Table D-2. Alternative Calculation of Average Costs for All of VHA's Health Care Provided to OCO Patients (Dollars)

Treatment Group	Treatment Year 1	Treatment Year 2	Treatment Year 3	Treatment Year 4
PTSD or TBI				
PTSD[a]	8,300	5,200	5,100	5,100
TBI[b]	11,700	6,000	10,800	18,300
Both PTSD and TBI	13,800	8,900	9,300	10,200
No PTSD or TBI	2,400	2,300	2,300	2,300

Source: Congressional Budget Office based on data from the Department of Veterans Affairs, Veterans Health Administration.

Notes: Data cover fiscal years 2004 to 2009 for up to the first four years of treatment. Data exclude about 500 patients, many with PTSD and TBI, who entered VHA at Polytrauma Rehabilitation Centers.

Average annual costs are based on the number of OCO patients who sought treatment in a given year.

VHA converted costs provided to CBO to fiscal year 2009 dollars based on annual increases in the average cost of a primary care visit from 2004 to 2009. CBO then indexed those costs to 2011 dollars using the GDP deflator.

VHA = Veterans Health Administration; OCO = overseas contingency operations; PTSD = post-traumatic stress disorder; TBI = traumatic brain injury.

[a] Patients in the PTSD group did not have TBI, but many had other conditions.

[b] Patients in the TBI group did not have PTSD, but many had other conditions.

End Notes

[1] Diagnosis of mild TBI with persistent symptoms is complicated because the condition does not have a clinically validated definition—that is, a definition that is based on a substantive body of empirical research and is broadly accepted by the medical community. Moreover, many other conditions cause symptoms that are similar to those of mild TBI.

[2] All of the TBI patients in the data that CBO examined had symptomatic TBI—that is, they exhibited symptoms that were attributed to TBI at the time of VHA's medical screening or examination.

[3] VHA's clinical practices for TBI changed during the data period (2004 to 2009): In 2007, the agency initiated comprehensive screening for mild, symptomatic TBI. Therefore, patients whom VHA diagnosed with TBI in 2007 or later were more likely to have had mild TBI than those diagnosed before that year. As a result, the data that CBO analyzed included a smaller share of patients with mild TBI in their third and fourth years of treatment than in their first and second years. Because treating patients with moderate or severe TBI requires more extensive services and resources than does treating patients with mild TBI, that difference elevated the estimated average costs of treatment for TBI patients in the third and fourth years.

[4] For a recent overview of those costs, see the statement of Heidi L. W. Golding, Principal Analyst for Military and Veterans' Compensation, Congressional Budget Office, before the Senate Committee on Veterans' Affairs, *Potential Costs of Health Care for Veterans of Recent and Ongoing U.S. Military Operations* (July 27, 2011).

[5] Defense and Veterans Brain Injury Center, TBI Facts, accessed June 27, 2011, at www.dvbic.org/TBI---The-Military/ TBI-Facts.aspx.

[6] For further discussion, see Susanne Meares and others, "The Prospective Course of Postconcussion Syndrome: The Role of Mild Traumatic Brain Injury," *Neuropsychology*, vol. 25, no. 4 (July 2011), pp. 1–12; and Charles W. Hoge and others, "Care of War Veterans with Mild Traumatic Brain Injury—Flawed Perspectives," *New England Journal of Medicine*, vol. 360, no. 16 (April 16, 2009), pp. 1588–1591.

[7] The largest category of diagnoses—diseases of the musculoskeletal system or connective tissue system—applied to 56 percent of OCO patients. Veterans may receive diagnoses in more than one category, so the percentages of patients with different diagnoses sum to more than 100 percent.

[8] The screen for deployment-related health risks includes questions designed to detect depression, alcohol abuse, and TBI, in addition to those relating to PTSD. The screen may be given in one of several venues but commonly occurs during a primary care visit.

[9] In addition to providing clinical care services, VHA operates about 300 Vet Centers for veterans and their families at no out-of-pocket cost. Vet Centers offer readjustment services such as individual and family counseling, assistance in applying for VHA benefits, and information on other community and educational opportunities. Veterans using those services need not be enrolled for VHA's health care services, and they retain anonymity for any counseling they receive.

[10] For more information, see VHA's National Center for PTSD Web site at www.ptsd.va.gov/public/index.asp.

[11] Institute of Medicine, *Treatment of Posttraumatic Stress Disorder: An Assessment of the Evidence* (Washington, D.C.: National Academies Press, 2008).

[12] Karen Seal and others, "VA Mental Health Services Utilization in Iraq and Afghanistan Veterans in the First Year of Receiving New Mental Health Diagnoses," *Journal of Traumatic Stress*, vol. 23, no. 1 (February 2010), pp. 5–16.

[13] Ibid.

[14] Michele R. Spoont and others, "Treatment Receipt by Veterans After a PTSD Diagnosis in PTSD, Mental Health, or General Medical Clinics," *Psychiatric Services*, vol. 61, no. 1 (January 2010), pp. 58–63.

[15] David Cifu, National Director of VA's Physical Medicine and Rehabilitation Office, "The Veterans Health Administration Poly-trauma System of Care" (PowerPoint slides transmitted via e-mail, May 2010).There is some controversy surrounding estimates of the prevalence of symptomatic TBI. Headaches, concentration and memory problems, fatigue, irritability, and sleep disturbance are common symptoms seen in veterans returning from war, as well as in individuals with other medical conditions. Whether symptoms that occur months or years after a TBI can be unequivocally attributed to mild TBI, as opposed to other conditions, has been the subject of considerable debate. See Charles Hoge and others, "Care of War Veterans with Mild Traumatic Brain Injury—Flawed Perspectives," *New England Journal of Medicine*, vol. 360 (April 16, 2009), pp. 1588–1591.

[16] For a more extensive discussion of the challenges that VHA clinicians face in diagnosing TBI, see Heather Belanger and others, "The Veterans Health Administration's System of Care for Mild Traumatic Brain Injury: Costs, Benefits, and Controversies," *Journal of Head Trauma Rehabilitation*, vol. 24, no. 1 (2009), pp.4–13.

[17] Information presented in this and the following paragraph is from a document prepared jointly by the Department of Veterans Affairs and the Department of Defense, *VA/DoD Clinical Practice Guideline for Management of Concussion/Mild Traumatic Brain Injury*, April 2009.

[18] Institute of Medicine, *Gulf War and Health,* vol. 7, *Long-Term Consequences of Traumatic Brain Injury* (Washington, D.C.: National Academies Press, 2009).

[19] Another study reported that among soldiers who had just returned from a deployment to Iraq, about one-third who reported suffering a mild TBI also screened positive for PTSD. See Lisa Brenner and others, "Traumatic Brain Injury, Posttraumatic Stress Disorder, and Postconcussive Symptoms: Symptom Reporting Among Troops Returning from Iraq," *Journal of Head Trauma Rehabilitation*, vol. 25, no. 5 (September-October 2010), pp. 307–312. There is some evidence that PTSD explains most or all symptoms in OCO veterans with concussions. See Charles W. Hoge and others, "Mild Traumatic Brain Injury in U.S. Soldiers Returning from Iraq," *New England Journal of Medicine*, vol. 358, no. 5 (January 31, 2008), pp. 453–463.

[20] The five centers are located in Minneapolis, Minn.; Palo Alto, Calif.; Richmond, Va.; Tampa, Fla.; and San Antonio, Tex. For more information, see VHA's Polytrauma/TBI System of Care Web site at www.polytrauma.va.gov.

[21] VHA, for example, created a Mental Health Enhancement Initiative to provide funding to facilitate greater community outreach, place PTSD specialists or treatment teams in each VHA Medical Center, and expand evidence-based care for PTSD.

[22] The Wounded, Ill, and Injured Senior Oversight Committee is among numerous review groups, task forces, and commissions that have examined or are currently charged with improving the care and benefits that DoD and VA provide to service members and veterans.

[23] Government Accountability Office, *DOD and VA Have Jointly Developed the Majority of Required Policies but Challenges Remain,* GAO-09-728 (July 2009).

[24] The Defense and Veterans Brain Injury Center became one of the component centers of the Defense Centers of Excellence for Psychological Health and Traumatic Brain Injury, an umbrella organization that was established in November 2007. For more information, see the Defense Centers of Excellence Web site at www.dcoe.health.

[25] Robin M. Weinick and others, *Programs Addressing Psychological Health and Traumatic Brain Injury Among U.S. Military Service-members and Their Families* (Santa Monica, Calif.: RAND Corporation, 2011).

[26] NwHIN is led by the Department of Health and Human Services. For more information, see http://healthit.hhs.gov/portal/server.pt/ community/healthit_hhs_gov nhin_exchange/1407.

[27] VHA did not provide CBO with data from the start of overseas contingency operations in 2001. However, the number of OCO veterans entering VHA before 2004 was relatively small: Roughly 10,000 veterans who deployed to Iraq and Afghanistan had sought VHA's health care services by the end of 2003.

[28] Vet Centers provided PTSD services to 42,000 OCO veterans through June 2011; among those veterans, 27,000 were also seen for PTSD at a VHA medical center. The data that CBO analyzed do not include information on the 15,000 veterans seen only at Vet Centers.

[29] In the information that it provided to CBO, VHA converted its cost data to fiscal year 2009 dollars on the basis of annual increases in the average cost of a primary care visit from 2004 to 2009. CBO then indexed those costs to 2011 dollars using the implicit price deflator for gross domestic product.

[30] Initial hospitalizations for the more severe cases of TBI are not included in VHA's costs because those individuals were still on active duty at the time of initial injury and would have been treated within DoD.

[31] TBI describes an injury event, but the term TBI may also refer to symptoms that persist beyond the acute period. In this study, TBI patients are OCO veterans who, when examined at VHA facilities, exhibited symptoms attributed to a TBI.

[32] To determine the group to which a patient belonged, each OCO patient's administrative record was checked for any diagnosis code of PTSD or TBI, and the patient was assigned to the relevant group. Any patient with both codes was classified as having both PTSD and TBI. No patient could be included in more than one diagnosis group; once classified, patients remained in the same group for the entire sample period. The sample included all PTSD and TBI cases among OCO veterans diagnosed at VHA, regardless of whether those conditions were sustained while deployed. The share of veterans who acquired PTSD or TBI unrelated to deployment (for example, injury from an automobile accident after returning from Iraq or Afghanistan) is unknown but is probably a small portion of CBO's sample.

[33] Veterans who became part of CBO's sample in those later years are more likely to have remained in the military longer after deployment than those who entered in the early years of 2004 and 2005. Any health conditions that veterans who entered VHA in 2008 and 2009 developed during deployment, therefore, were more likely to have been treated by DoD before those service members transferred to VHA. The extension of enhanced eligibility in 2008 appears to have had a minimal effect on entry into the VHA system. VHA provided CBO with data showing that both before and after the policy change, most veterans who used VHA services did so within two years of separation from active duty.

[34] VHA computes costs on the basis of its internal reporting systems. Costs for treating PTSD and TBI in the civilian population and veterans treated at VHA are unlikely to be comparable because of differences in cost allocation methodologies, the populations treated, and the mechanisms of injury. Also, while VHA data measure the costs of care, private-sector estimates are often based on insurance reimbursements to private providers, which are not identical to costs.

[35] VHA researchers examining OCO veterans treated at VHA have reported rates of concurrent diagnoses that are similar to CBO's; however, some researchers drawing from broader samples of OCO service members and veterans find lower rates of concurrent TBI and PTSD. In the three studies with the largest sample sizes, between 33 percent and 39 percent of OCO veterans with mild TBI also screened positive for PTSD. See Kathleen F. Carlson and others, "Prevalence, Assessment, and Treatment of Mild Traumatic Brain Injury and Posttraumatic Stress Disorder: A Systematic Review of the Evidence," *Journal of Head Trauma Rehabilitation*, vol. 26, no. 2 (March–April 2011), pp. 103–115.

[36] If the threshold is raised to include only veterans who had two or more visits coded with a diagnosis of PTSD or TBI, the rates that CBO estimates drop to 20 percent and 3 percent, respectively. (Some researchers consider a

two-visit measure a more definitive indicator of a condition, although that more-stringent threshold will miss those veterans who have PTSD or TBI but leave the VHA system after the initial diagnosis.)

[37] Those studies included papers that reported frequencies of possible cases of PTSD or TBI regardless of whether the objective of the study was to estimate the prevalence in the broader OCO population.

[38] For a discussion of future spending on health care for OCO veterans, see Congressional Budget Office, *Potential Costs of Veterans' Health Care* (October 2010).

[39] Veterans enrolled in the VHA system usually have other sources of health care available to them and use VHA's services for a minority of their care. Because CBO has no data on OCO veterans' use of health care outside of VHA, it cannot determine differences in the total health care services used by the different groups. Consequently, OCO veterans with no diagnosis of PTSD or TBI may receive a higher or lower portion of their care from VHA than the other groups.

[40] Inpatient care includes medical or surgical care, rehabilitation medicine, residential rehabilitation, inpatient PTSD care, inpatient psychiatric care, PTSD residential rehabilitation, and nursing home care. Because only one or two categories of inpatient care generally accounted for a substantial share of treatment, only the largest categories are reported here.

[41] Outpatient care includes care provided in various types of clinics: primary care, medical/surgical care, mental health, PTSD, TBI, polytrauma, and a more general type denoted as "other." Diagnostic tests are also included in outpatient care. Because only one or two categories of outpatient care typically accounted for a substantial share of treatment, only the largest categories are reported here.

[42] The number of prescriptions filled includes the dispensing of pharmaceuticals and over-the-counter drugs (as measured in 30-day equivalents), as well as related supplies.

[43] See Appendix B for a description of CBO's methodology. VHA has reported the number of OCO patients and their associated costs in the various editions of the agency's annual budget documentation. VHA treated 508,000 OCO veterans from 2002 through 2009. The data that VHA supplied to CBO encompassed 98 percent of that population and, because some overhead costs were not included, about 92 percent of the total costs.

[44] By contrast, VHA projects that spending per veteran user for all eras will be an estimated $9,100 in 2011.

[45] In the data provided to CBO, TBI patients who used VHA's services for four years were diagnosed before 2007, when VHA began comprehensive screening of OCO veterans for mild TBI. Consequently, the portion of the sample drawn before 2007 was much smaller and probably included relatively more cases of moderate or severe TBI than later cohorts, making costs for patients with four treatment years unreliable in predicting future spending.

[46] If diagnostic and pharmacy costs were excluded, the average costs would be approximately 20 percent to 35 percent lower than reported here.

[47] Reliable, up-to-date estimates of the total costs of PTSD and TBI are not available for the general population. In addition, cost estimates for civilians would not be comparable to those for the military partly because the mechanism of injury is different. Among OCO veterans, most TBIs are the result of explosions; military PTSD is typically related to combat.

[48] Ann Hendricks and others, "Screening for Mild Traumatic Brain Injury in OEF/OIF Deployed Military: An Empirical Assessment of the VHA Experience," (paper presented at the National Conference of VA's Health Services Research and Development Service, Washington, D.C., February 16–18, 2011).

[49] Brent Taylor and others, "Prevalence and Costs of Co-Occurring TBI, Psychiatric Disturbance, and Pain Among OEF/OEF VA Users," (paper presented at the National Conference of VA's Health Services Research and Development Service, Washington, D.C., February 16–18, 2011).

[50] In RAND's *Invisible Wounds of War*, researchers estimated the 2005 societal costs, including the costs from unemployment and suicide, of treating service members who deployed to overseas contingency operations. The researchers found that the costs of PTSD ranged from $5,900 to $10,300 for two years.

Using Medicare reimbursement rates and other data, the researchers reported that the societal costs of TBI for one year ranged from $26,000 to $31,000 for mild cases and from $252,000 to $383,000 for moderate and severe cases. Because the data undercounted the number of mild TBIs and overcounted the number of hospitalizations attributable to those mild cases, the reported costs for mild TBI are likely to be substantially overstated. RAND's estimates of societal costs should not be compared with CBO's numbers, which focus only on VHA's costs.

(Unlike RAND's estimates, CBO's estimates of the costs of treating TBI exclude the initial hospitalizations of the more severe cases because those individuals were still on active duty at the time of initial injury and hospitalization and therefore would have been treated within DoD.) See Terri Tanielian and Lisa H. Jaycox, eds., *Invisible Wounds of War: Psychological and Cognitive Injuries, Their Consequences, and Services to Assist Recovery* (Santa Monica, Calif.: RAND Corporation, 2008).

[51] Because polytrauma patients have many other medical conditions, it is difficult to attribute a portion of their total costs of care specifically to PTSD and TBI. The relatively high average costs credited to PTSD- and TBI-specific care is probably an artifact of how such costs are allocated. See Appendix B.

End Notes for Appendix A

[1] For more detail, see the *Diagnostic and Statistical Manual of Mental Disorders* (DSM), 4th ed., rev. (Arlington, Va.: American Psychiatric Publishing, 2000). In previous editions, the DSM required that the trauma be outside the range of usual human experience but set no requirement for impairment. More recently, according to the committee revising the DSM, the requirement that the trauma result in horror, fear, or helplessness may be eliminated in the 5th edition of the DSM, scheduled for release in 2013.

[2] Information for this section was compiled from the following sources: Institute of Medicine, *Gulf War and Health*, vol. 6, *Physiologic, Psychologic, and Psychosocial Effects of Deployment-Related Stress* (Washington, D.C.: National Academies Press, 2008); J.D. Bremner and others, "Chronic PTSD in Vietnam Combat Veterans: Course of Illness and Substance Abuse, *American Journal of Psychiatry*, vol. 153, no. 3 (1996), pp. 369–375; Naomi Breslau and others, "Trauma and Posttraumatic Stress Disorder in the Community," *Archives of General Psychiatry*, vol. 55, (July 1998), pp. 626–632; Naomi Breslau, "Outcomes of Posttraumatic Stress Disorder," *Journal of Clinical Psychiatry*, vol. 62, supplement 17 (2001), pp. 55–59; Ronald C. Kessler and others, "Posttraumatic Stress Disorder in the National Comorbidity Survey," *Archives of General Psychiatry*, vol. 52 (December 1995), pp. 1048–1060; Kathryn M. Connor and Marian I. Butterfield, "Posttraumatic Stress Disorder," *Focus*, vol. 1, no. 3 (Summer 2003), pp. 247– 261; and Paula P. Schnurr and others, "A Descriptive Analysis of PTSD Chronicity in Vietnam Veterans," *Journal of Traumatic Stress*, vol. 16, no. 6 (December 2003), pp. 545–553; Karestan C. Koenen and others, "Risk Factors for Course of Posttraumatic Stress Disorder Among Vietnam Veterans: A 14-Year Follow-Up of American Legionnaires," *Journal of Consulting and Clinical Psychology*, vol. 71, no. 6 (2003), pp. 980–986.

[3] For a more detailed discussion about risk and protective factors, see Institute of Medicine, *Gulf War and Health*, vol. 6, *Physiologic, Psychologic, and Psychosocial Effects of Deployment-Related Stress.*

[4] Department of Health and Human Services, Centers for Disease Control and Prevention, National Center for Injury Prevention and Control, *Traumatic Brain Injury in the United States: A Report to Congress* (December 1999).

[5] T. Kay and others, "Definition of Mild Traumatic Brain Injury," *Journal of Head Trauma Rehabilitation*, vol. 8, no. 3 (September 1993), pp. 86–87. Criteria by the Department of Veterans Affairs and the Department of Defense for severity are largely consistent with the above guidance, although they have one additional criterion for mild TBI: Brain imaging results must be normal. Service members who meet the other criteria for mild TBI but have abnormal brain imaging results are rated as having moderate TBIs.

Service members who meet the criteria for more than one severity level are rated at the higher severity. See Department of Veterans Affairs and Department of Defense, *VA/DOD Clinical Practice Guideline for Management of Concussion/Mild Traumatic Brain Injury*, April 2009.

[6] The DSM-IV and ICD-10 (*International Classification of Diseases*, 10th ed.) define the condition differently, which often results in diagnostic disagreement. In addition, controversy surrounds the diagnosis of the condition—specifically, whether symptoms that occur after an injury can be unequivocally attributed to mild TBI, as opposed to other conditions.

See Corwin Boake and others, "Diagnostic Criteria for Postconcussional Syndrome After Mild to Moderate Traumatic Brain Injury," *Journal of Neuropsychiatry and Clinical Neuroscience,* vol. 17, no. 3 (Summer 2005), pp. 350–356; and Linda J. Carroll and others, "Methodological Issues and Research Recommendations for Mild Traumatic Brain Injury: The WHO Collaborating Centre Task Force on Mild Traumatic Brain Injury," *Journal of Rehabilitation Medicine*, vol. 36, supplement 43 (February 2004), pp. 113–125. The Department of Veterans Affairs and the Department of Defense's clinical guidelines for diagnosing and treating mild TBI do not endorse either the DSM's or ICD's definition of PCS.

[7] For more information on the effects of TBI, see Institute of Medicine, *Gulf War and Health*, vol. 7, *Long-Term Consequences of Traumatic Brain Injury* (National Academies Press: Washington, D.C., 2008).

[8] See Linda J. Carroll and others, "Prognosis for Mild Traumatic Brain Injury: Results of the WHO Collaborating Centre Task Force on Mild Traumatic Brain Injury," *Journal of Rehabilitation Medicine*, vol. 36, supplement 43 (February 2004), pp. 84–105; Heather G. Belanger and others, "The Veterans Health Administration System of Care for Mild Traumatic Brain Injury: Costs, Benefits, and Controversies," *Journal of Head Trauma Rehabilitation*, vol. 24, no. 1 (January–February 2009), pp. 4–13; Charles Hoge and others, "Care of War Veterans with Mild Traumatic Brain Injury—Flawed Perspectives," *New England Journal of Medicine*, vol. 360 (April 16, 2009), pp. 1588–1591.

[9] See Carroll and others, "Prognosis for Mild Traumatic Brain Injury"; Michael P. Alexander, "Mild Traumatic Brain Injury: Pathophysiology, Natural History, and Clinical Management," *Neurology*, vol. 45, no. 7 (July 1995), pp. 1253–1260; and Thomas W. McAllister, "Mild Brain Injury and the Post-concussion Syndrome," in Jonathan M. Silver, Thomas W. McAllister, and Stuart C. Yudofsky, eds., *Textbook of Traumatic Brain Injury* (Arlington, Va.: American Psychiatric Publishing, 2004), pp. 279–309.

[10] See Michael A. McCrea, *Mild Traumatic Brain Injury and Postconcussion Syndrome: The New Evidence Base for Diagnosis and Treatment* (New York: Oxford University Press, 2008); Alexander, "Mild Traumatic Brain Injury," pp. 1253–1260; Heather G. Belanger and others, "Factors Moderating Neuropsychological Outcomes Following Mild Traumatic Brain Injury: A Meta-Analysis," *Journal of the International Neuropsychological Society*, vol. 11, no. 3 (2005), pp. 215–227; and Grant L. Iverson, "Outcome from Mild Traumatic Brain Injury," *Current Opinion in Psychiatry*, vol. 18, no. 3 (May 2005), pp. 301–317.

[11] See Heather Belanger and others, "The Veterans Health Administration System of Care for Mild Traumatic Brain Injury: Costs, Benefits, and Controversies"; also see Carroll and others, "Prognosis for Mild Traumatic Brain Injury."

End Notes for Appendix B

[1] Because of small sample sizes for female veterans and some age groups, CBO does not report analyses along those dimensions.

[2] Although some researchers have used Medicare reimbursement data to estimate health care costs, those data would not have been useful for CBO's analysis, which focuses solely on VHA's costs. VHA's costs and Medicare reimbursement rates are structurally different and therefore not directly comparable. As a health insurance system, Medicare reimburses providers on the basis of a price schedule for various services classified by diagnosis codes; negotiated prices presumably reflect the providers' costs, but they are not equal to those costs. By contrast, VHA is a direct health care provider with an accounting system designed to measure the direct and indirect costs of each health care encounter. In addition, services are not necessarily comparable. For example, VHA hospital stays include the costs of services provided by physicians; by contrast, Medicare's reimbursements to hospitals for inpatient stays do not.

End Notes for Appendix C

[1] The range includes studies that reported frequencies of PTSD regardless of whether the study objective was to estimate the prevalence in a population of service members or veterans. For a survey of the literature, see Rajeev Ramchand and others, "Disparate Prevalence Estimates of PTSD Among Service Members Who Served in Iraq and Afghanistan: Possible Explanations," *Journal of Traumatic Stress*, vol. 23, no. 1 (February 2010), pp. 59–68.

[2] Richard A. Kulka and others, *The National Vietnam Veterans Readjustment Study: Tables of Findings and Technical Appendices* (New York: Brunner/Mazel, 1990); and Richard A. Kulka and others, *Trauma and the Vietnam War Generation: Report of Findings from the National Vietnam Veterans Readjustment Study* (New York: Brunner/Mazel, 1990).

[3] Bruce Dohrenwend and others, "The Psychological Risks of Vietnam for U.S. Veterans: A Revisit with New Data and Methods," *Science*, vol. 313, no. 979 (August 18, 2006), pp. 979–982. The diagnostic tool and methodology used in the reanalysis of the NVRRS differed from those used in the earlier study. The change in the diagnostic tool alone reduced the estimated prevalence of PTSD by 3 percentage points. Adjusting for

changes in the clinical definition of PTSD and using additional data from personnel records decreased the prevalence rate an additional 3 percentage points.

[4] For example, recent veterans are more likely to have completed high school than were draftees during the Vietnam War. Also, American society may be more supportive of its returning service members now than it was during the Vietnam War.

[5] Researchers may use different methods to determine whether an individual screens positive using the PCL. Under the cluster method, personnel screened positive if they reported at least one intrusion symptom, three avoidance symptoms, and two hyper-arousal symptoms at the moderate level or higher. An alternate method requires assigning a number to the severity of each symptom ("not at all" = 0 points through "extremely bothered" = 5 points). To screen positive for PTSD, a score of at least 50 on a scale of 17 to 85 is often required.

[6] Terri Tanielian and Lisa Jaycox, eds., *Invisible Wounds of War: Psychological and Cognitive Injuries, Their Consequences, and Services to Assist Recovery,* (Santa Monica, Calif.: RAND Corporation, 2008).

[7] Tyler C. Smith and others, "New Onset and Persistent Symptoms of Post-Traumatic Stress Disorder Self Reported After Deployment and Combat Exposures: Prospective Population Based U.S. Military Cohort Study," *British Medical Journal,* vol. 336, no. 7640 (February 16, 2008), pp. 366–371.

[8] Upon service members' completion of their deployment, DoD administers the four-question Primary Care PTSD screen (PCPTSD) in the Post-Deployment Health Assessment and, again, generally three to six months later, in the Post-Deployment Health Reassessment.

[9] Charles S. Milliken and others, "Longitudinal Assessment of Mental Health Problems Among Active and Reserve Component Soldiers Returning from the Iraq War," *Journal of the American Medical Association,* vol. 298, no. 18 (November 14, 2007), pp. 2141–2148. The prevalence estimates presented in that study are based on the DoD-administered Post-Deployment Health Assessment. The range in rates is the result of two alternate methods for determining PTSD: The lower rate reflects service members' endorsement of three or more symptom clusters from the four-item screening instrument, and the higher rate reflects the positive endorsement of two or more symptom clusters.

[10] For example, the PCL (17-item checklist) and the PC-PTSD (four-item screen) do not explicitly establish significant distress or impairment in social, occupational, or other areas of functioning. In addition, the PCL does not ask whether the person was exposed to a traumatic event.

[11] Milliken presented data using two thresholds: answering positively to two or more questions and, alternatively, to three or more questions on the four-question PC-PTSD. Using the higher threshold almost halved (to 6 percent) the number of PTSD cases for active Army soldiers immediately after deployment.

[12] A 2004 study by Annabel Prins and others estimated that the PC-PTSD had a sensitivity of 0.77 and a specificity of 0.85 using a three-out-of-four question threshold. Those values imply that 77 percent of service members with PTSD screen positive (sensitivity equals 0.77), and 15 percent of those without the disease also screen positive (specificity equals 0.85). CBO estimates that, if the true population prevalence is 15 percent and 1,000 people are screened, a total of 244 people (24 percent) would be expected to test positive: 116 of the 150 people (77 percent) who have the disease, and 128 of the 850 people (15 percent) who do not (the false positives). In that case, the rate of screening positive is about 60 percent higher than the true prevalence of the disease. See Annabel Prins and others, "The Primary Care PTSD Screen (PC-PTSD): Development and Operating Characteristics: Corrigendum," *Primary Care Psychiatry*, vol. 9, no. 4 (2004), p. 151; Artin Terhakopian and others, "Estimating Population Prevalence of Posttraumatic Stress Disorder: An Example Using the PTSD Checklist," *Journal of Traumatic Stress*, vol. 21, no. 3 (June 2008), pp. 290–300; and Heidi Golding and others, "Understanding Recent Estimates of PTSD and TBI from Operations Iraqi Freedom and Enduring Freedom," *Journal of Rehabilitation Research and Development*, vol. 46, no. 5 (2009), pp. vii–xiii.

[13] One study by McLay and others illustrates that type of reporting problem. Using a sample of medical personnel within the Department of Defense, the study found that delivering the PCL anonymously generated double the rate of positive PTSD cases than found in PCL results that become part of a service member's medical record. However, generalizing those results is problematic because the respondents to the anonymous screen were a small subset of the larger population and may not have been representative. See Robert N. McLay and others, "On-the-Record Screenings Versus Anonymous Surveys in Reporting PTSD," *American Journal of Psychiatry*, vol. 165, no. 6 (June 2008), pp. 775–776.

[14] Charles W. Hoge and others, "Mild Traumatic Brain Injury in U.S. Soldiers Returning from Iraq." *New England Journal of Medicine*, vol. 358, no. 5 (January 31, 2008), pp. 453–463.

[15] Tanielian and Jaycox, eds., *Invisible Wounds of War.*

[16] Heidi Terrio and others, "Traumatic Brain Injury Screening: Preliminary Findings in a U.S. Army Brigade Combat Team," *Journal of Head Trauma Rehabilitation*, vol. 24, no. 1 (January– February 2009), pp. 14–23.

[17] Ann Hendricks and others, "Screening for Mild Traumatic Brain Injury in OEF-OIF Deployed Military: An Empirical Assessment of the VHA Experience" (paper presented at the National Conference of VA's Health Services Research and Development Service, Washington, D.C., February 2011).

[18] To view the questionnaire, see "3 Question DVBIC TBI Screening Tool Instruction Sheet," available at www.dvbic.org/images/ pdfs/3-Question-Screening-Tool.aspx. That screening tool asks service members to identify injuries that occurred during deployment by certain mechanisms such as an explosion or a fall; it asks whether any injuries resulted in a change in consciousness, such as "seeing stars," immediately following the event; and it also asks the respondents, "Are you currently experiencing any of the following problems that you think might be related to a possible head injury or concussion?" It does not ask whether symptoms may be related to other causes. RAND researchers considered the test positive for TBI if the individual endorsed any of the injuries listed in the first question and reported any alteration of consciousness detailed in the second question. Terrio used the same screening criteria but followed up with a clinical assessment. Hoge queried soldiers on a smaller set of changes in consciousness than the BTBIS offers.

[19] Kerry T. Donnelly and others, "Reliability, Sensitivity, and Specificity of the VA Traumatic Brain Injury Screening Tool," *Journal of Head Trauma Rehabilitation,* vol. 26, no. 6 (November– December 2011), pp. 439–453; also see Karen A. Schwab and others, "Screening for Traumatic Brain Injury in Troops Returning from Deployment in Afghanistan and Iraq: Initial Investigation of the Usefulness of a Short Screening Tool for Traumatic Brain Injury," *Journal of Head Trauma Rehabilitation*, vol. 22, no. 6 (November-December 2007), pp. 377–389.

[20] One study found that the self-reported concussion rate was 9 percent about one month before soldiers returned home from deployment but jumped to 22 percent when the same sample was surveyed one year after deployment. See Melissa A. Polusny and others, "Longitudinal Effects of Mild Traumatic Brain Injury and Posttraumatic Stress Disorder Comorbidity on Postdeployment Outcomes in National Guard Soldiers Deployed to Iraq," *Archives of General Psychiatry*, vol. 68, no. 1 (January 2011), pp. 79–89.

[21]See Heather Belanger and others, "The Veterans Health Administration System of Care for Mild Traumatic Brain Injury: Costs, Benefits, and Controversies," *Journal of Head Trauma Rehabilitation*, vol. 24, no. 1 (2009), pp. 4–13; also see Charles W. Hoge and others, "Care of War Veterans with Mild Traumatic Brain Injury—Flawed Perspectives," *New England Journal of Medicine*, vol. 360, no. 16 (April 16, 2009), pp. 1588–1591.

In: Treatment of PTSD and Traumatic Brain Injury ... ISBN: 978-1-62081-689-9
Editors: Aiden D. Thomas and Milton L. Harris

Chapter 2

DEPARTMENT OF DEFENSE: USE OF NEUROCOGNITIVE ASSESSMENT TOOLS IN POST-DEPLOYMENT IDENTIFICATION OF MILD TRAUMATIC BRAIN INJURY*

United States Government Accountability Office

Traumatic brain injury (TBI) has emerged as a serious concern among U.S. forces serving in military operations in Afghanistan and Iraq. The widespread use of improvised explosive devices in these conflicts increases the likelihood that servicemembers will sustain a TBI, which the Department of Defense (DOD) defines as a traumatically induced structural injury and/or physiological disruption of brain function as a result of an external force.[1] TBI cases within DOD are generally classified as mild, moderate, severe, or penetrating. From 2000 to March 2011 there were a total of 212,742 TBI cases reported by the Defense and Veterans Brain Injury Center within DOD. A majority of these cases, 163,181, were classified as mild traumatic brain injuries (mTBI)—commonly referred to as concussions.[2]

Early detection of injury is critical in TBI patient management. Diagnosis of moderate and severe TBI usually occurs in a timely manner due to the obvious and visible nature of the head injury. Identification of mTBI presents a challenge due to its less obvious nature. With mTBI, there may be no observable head injury. In addition, in the combat theater, an mTBI may not be identified if it occurs at the same time as other combat injuries that are more visible or life-threatening, such as orthopedic injuries or open wounds. Furthermore, some of the symptoms of mTBI—such as irritability and insomnia—are similar to those associated with other conditions, such as post-traumatic stress disorder.

Although the majority of patients with mTBI recover quickly with minimal intervention, a subset of patients develops lingering symptoms that interfere with social and occupational functioning. Accurate and timely identification of mTBI is important as treatment can mitigate the physical, emotional, and cognitive effects of the injury. Neurocognitive deficits associated

* This is an edited, reformatted and augmented version of United States Government Accountability Office, Publication No. GAO-12-27R, dated October 24, 2011.

with mTBI can be identified by neurocognitive assessment tools. These tools generally consist of a series of tests that measure cognitive performance areas that may be impaired by an mTBI such as attention, judgment, and memory.

Identification of mTBI in servicemembers who served in Afghanistan and Iraq has been the subject of recent media attention, with particular attention focused on the proper use of neurocognitive assessment tools to screen all servicemembers post-deployment for deficits or symptoms related to mTBI. In this context and in response to your request, this report describes (1) DOD's post-deployment policy on the use of neurocognitive assessment tools as a stand-alone initial screen to identify servicemembers who may have sustained an mTBI during deployment; (2) what informed DOD's decisions to establish this post-deployment policy; and (3) mTBI experts' views on the science related to DOD's policy decision.[3] Additionally, you have expressed the importance of recording mTBI in a servicemember's medical history to ensure proper treatment. In response to this concern, we are initiating a review of DOD's in-theater documentation of servicemembers involved in potentially concussive events.

To describe DOD's post-deployment policy on the use of neurocognitive assessment tools as a stand-alone initial screen to identify servicemembers who may have sustained an mTBI during deployment, and what informed DOD's decisions to establish this post-deployment policy, we reviewed relevant DOD policy and guidance and interviewed DOD officials involved in DOD TBI policy. We also reviewed documents that DOD cited as support for its decision, such as task force and expert panel reports, and scientific studies. To describe mTBI experts' views on the science related to the policy decision, we interviewed 15 mTBI experts within and outside of DOD in the fields of military concussion and sports concussion. We selected experts through a snowball sampling method and through structured searches of the military and sports concussion literature.[4] We interviewed sports concussion experts because the sports population has experience in the use of neurocognitive assessment tools to help identify mTBI. The views of the experts we interviewed cannot be assumed to be the views of all mTBI experts.

We conducted this performance audit from April 2011 through October 2011 in accordance with generally accepted government auditing standards. Those standards require that we plan and perform the audit to obtain sufficient, appropriate evidence to provide a reasonable basis for our findings and conclusions based on our audit objectives. We believe that the evidence obtained provides a reasonable basis for our findings and conclusions based on our audit objectives.

RESULTS IN BRIEF

DOD does not require that all servicemembers be screened post-deployment using a neurocognitive assessment tool but does require that all servicemembers be screened using a set of TBI screening questions. According to DOD officials, this policy was informed by findings and recommendations from several task forces and expert panel reports, and scientific studies. Additionally, mTBI experts told us that the scientific evidence supports DOD's policy. For example, these experts told us that neurocognitive assessment tools cannot determine whether low cognitive function is caused by an mTBI. These experts told us, however, that neurocognitive assessment tools can be useful as part of a full clinical evaluation for a person who has already screened positive for a possible mTBI.

DOD Policy Does Not Require Screening All Servicemembers with a Neurocognitive Assessment Tool Post-Deployment

DOD policy does not require that all servicemembers receive an assessment with a neurocognitive assessment tool as a stand-alone initial screen for mTBI post-deployment. Instead, DOD requires initial screening of all servicemembers using TBI screening questions as part of the post-deployment health assessment (PDHA) process. The PDHA process is designed to self-identify and refer for further evaluation servicemembers with health concerns as a result of deployment.[5] During the PDHA process, a servicemember completes a form that includes TBI screening questions.[6] A health care provider reviews the completed form and may refer the servicemember to a clinician for further evaluation for a possible mTBI.[7] As part of that evaluation, a DOD official told us that clinicians may choose, but are not required, to use a neurocognitive assessment tool to help identify symptoms consistent with an mTBI. DOD anticipates issuing in the first quarter of calendar year 2012 additional policy on post-deployment neurocognitive assessment tools, according to a DOD official. The DOD policy will specify the use of a particular tool that clinicians should use if they choose to use a neurocognitive assessment tool during the clinical evaluation of a servicemember referred post-deployment through the PDHA process.

A May 28, 2008, DOD interim guidance requires that neurocognitive assessments using the Automated Neuropsychological Assessment Metrics (ANAM) neurocognitive assessment tool be administered to all servicemembers prior to deployment. According to a DOD official, the upcoming policy on post-deployment neurocognitive assessment will also specify use of the ANAM, if clinicians choose to use a neurocognitive assessment tool. DOD is currently conducting a head-to-head study of five neurocognitive assessment tools (including the ANAM) in order to identify the tool best suited to military use. After significant delay, DOD anticipates results of that study in 2015. DOD officials told us that DOD will then specify that the selected tool be used consistent with DOD policy on neurocognitive assessment.

Reports and Scientific Studies Informed DOD's Policy

According to a DOD official with responsibility for DOD's policy on mTBI, the use of neurocognitive assessment tools post-deployment was informed by findings and recommendations from several task forces and expert panel reports, and scientific studies.

The DOD official told us that DOD determined that these sources did not provide evidence to support the use of neurocognitive assessment tools as a standalone initial screen for mTBI for all servicemembers post-deployment. The DOD official cited several reports as supporting their policy of not requiring that all servicemembers be assessed with a neurocognitive assessment tool post-deployment because these reports are silent on the use of such tools postdeployment.[8]

Additionally, the DOD official told us that one report and two scientific studies provided further support for not using a neurocognitive assessment tool as a stand-alone initial screen for mTBI for all servicemembers when they return from deployment.

The following describes the recommendation and suggestions of the report and studies and the DOD official's explanation of how they provided support for DOD's policy.

- The 2007 Army TBI Task Force report to the Surgeon General[9] recommended that DOD implement a post-deployment neuropsychological evaluation using the ANAM. However, the report reiterated several limitations of using a neurocognitive assessment tool as a stand-alone initial screen for mTBI, including limitations that could affect the accuracy of the tool.
  The DOD official told us that the report's recommendation in conjunction with the limitations regarding the use of neurocognitive assessment tools stated in the report supports their policy of using the PDHA, rather than the ANAM.
- A study conducted at Fort Bragg and published in 2009[10] found no association between poor ANAM performance after deployment and self-reported history of mTBI.
  The DOD official told us that this study provides evidence that screening all servicemembers post-deployment with a neurocognitive assessment tool is not likely to be useful.
- DOD has stated that findings from a study conducted at Ft. Campbell[11] support a selective use of the ANAM post-deployment but not as a stand-alone initial screen for mTBI for all servicemembers. The study found that at post-deployment, servicemembers reporting a history of mTBI, but not current mTBI symptoms, did not show a decline in cognitive functioning as measured by the ANAM.
  The DOD official told us that using the ANAM as a stand-alone initial screen for mTBI can result in false negative results for these servicemembers because the assessment tool was not able to identify that an mTBI had occurred for servicemembers without symptoms at post-deployment.[12]

MTBI Experts Told Us the Science Supports DOD's Policy

Experts in mTBI told us that the science related to neurocognitive assessment tools supports DOD's post-deployment policy with respect to screening for mTBI. These experts told us they do not believe that screening all servicemembers post-deployment with a neurocognitive assessment tool is beneficial to determine who may have sustained an mTBI during deployment. However, most of the experts told us they do believe that such tools can be useful to help a clinician determine whether a servicemember has sustained an mTBI in situations where a servicemember has already screened positive on the PDHA and was subsequently referred to a clinician for a full evaluation.

Experts gave several reasons why they support DOD's policy with respect to mTBI screening. For one, experts told us that neurocognitive assessment tools can indicate low cognitive function but cannot determine whether or not it is caused by an mTBI. They told us it is likely that confounding variables,[13] such as lack of sleep, stress, and influence of medication—not mTBI—can be the cause of change in cognition in servicemembers at post-deployment. They said that these confounding variables could result in a large number of false positives[14] when all servicemembers are assessed. Another reason is that such tools are designed to measure cognitive function and generally do not measure the physical aspects of mTBI, such as headaches, impaired balance, and sensitivity to light or noise. This oversight may potentially result in false negatives. Most experts told us that in order to reduce the number of false positives or negatives from assessments at post-deployment with a neurocognitive assessment tool, such tools should only be used during a full clinical evaluation for someone who already screened positive for the possibility of an mTBI on the PDHA. During that evaluation, the clinician can evaluate a servicemember's event history, symptoms, and cognitive functioning by means of a neurocognitive assessment tool to determine whether someone has sustained an mTBI.

A third reason experts gave for why they support DOD's policy involves the potential negative effect on the servicemember from a false positive outcome. Most experts told us that individuals who initially test positive for mTBI with a neurocognitive assessment tool—but after further evaluation are determined not to have sustained an mTBI—could still believe they sustained an mTBI and suffer lasting psychological effects from the initial false positive outcome. A few experts disagreed, saying an appropriate explanation by a clinician would likely mitigate any negative psychological effect of a false positive outcome.

AGENCY COMMENTS

We provided a draft of this report to DOD for comment. DOD concurred with our findings and provided written technical comments, which we incorporated as appropriate.

Randall B. Williamson
Director, Health Care

End Notes

[1] Department of Veterans Affairs/DOD, Clinical Practice Guideline for Management of Concussion/mild Traumatic Brain Injury (April 2009).

[2] DOD specifies that a person may be designated as having an mTBI only if the severity of the injury does not include: (1) loss of consciousness that lasted longer than 30 minutes; (2) alteration of consciousness for more than 24 hours; (3) post-traumatic amnesia lasting longer than 24 hours; or (4) an initial score of less than 13 on the Glasgow Coma Score, a widely-used 15-point scoring system for assessing coma and impaired consciousness. (Higher scores indicate a less severe injury while lower scores indicate a more severe injury.)

[3] For the purposes of this report, we define post-deployment as within 30 days after servicemembers' return from deployment.

[4] A snowball sample includes an initial list of cases, each of whom is asked for referrals to additional people, who are then interviewed and asked for referrals, and so on. We repeated this process until we were consistently receiving substantively similar information from each additional interview.

[5] DOD policy requires that the PDHA be completed by servicemembers within 30 days before or 30 days after return from deployment.

[6] The TBI screening questions on the PDHA are designed to be completed by the servicemember in four series. The sequence of questions specifically assesses (1) events that may have increased the risk of a TBI, (2) immediate symptoms following the event, (3) new or worsening symptoms following the event, and (4) current

symptoms. If there is a positive response to any question in the first series, the servicemember completes the second and third series; if there is a positive response to any question in the third series, the servicemember completes the fourth series about current symptoms. The form directs the health care provider to refer the servicemember based on the servicemember's current symptoms.

[7] According to the Department of Veterans Affairs/DOD Clinical Practice Guideline for Management of Concussion/mild Traumatic Brain Injury, a clinical evaluation for mTBI should include (1) obtaining a detailed medical history (including details of the injury event and identification of symptoms); (2) a psychosocial assessment (including assessment of conditions that may exacerbate mTBI symptoms, such as post-traumatic stress disorder); and (3) a physical exam.

[8] August 2006 report of the Armed Forces Epidemiology Board; April 2007 Independent Review Group on Rehabilitative Care and Administrative Processes at Walter Reed Army Medical Center and National Naval Medical Center; June 2007 report of the Defense Health Board Task Force on Mental Health; October 2007 report of the Scientific Advisory Panel on the Use of the ANAM; and Gulf War and Health: Volume 7: Long-Term Consequences of Traumatic Brain Injury, Committee on Gulf War and Health: Brain Injury in Veterans and Long-Term Health Outcomes (Institute of Medicine, 2008).

[9] Traumatic Brain Injury Task Force, Report to the Surgeon General (May 2007).

[10] Brian J. lvins, Robert Kane, Karen A. Schwab, "Performance on the Automated Neuropsychological Assessment Metrics in a Nonclinical Sample of Soldiers Screened for Mild TBI After Returning From Iraq and Afghanistan: A Descriptive Analysis," Journal of Head Trauma Rehabilitation, vol. 24, no. 1 (2009), 24-31.

[11] Tresa Roebuck-Spenser, Andrea S. Vincent, David A. Twille, Bret W. Logan, Mary Lopez, Stephen Grate, Robert E. Schlegel, Kirby Gilliland, Cognitive Change Associated with Deployment-Related Mild Traumatic Brain Injury Sustained During the OEF/OIF Conflicts. This is an unpublished manuscript provided to us by the Center for the Study of Human Operator Performance (C-SHOP) at the University of Oklahoma. The University of Oklahoma holds the license for ANAM technology.

[12] A false negative is an incorrect result of a diagnostic test or procedure that falsely indicates the absence of a finding, condition, or disease.

[13] A confounding variable is another variable that distorts the association being studied between the two main variables.

[14] A false positive is a test result that wrongly indicates the presence of a disease or other condition the test is designed to reveal.

In: Treatment of PTSD and Traumatic Brain Injury ... ISBN: 978-1-62081-689-9
Editors: Aiden D. Thomas and Milton L. Harris

Chapter 3

Management of Concussion/Mild Traumatic Brain Injury*

Department of Veterans Affairs
Department of Defense

Qualifying Statements

The Department of Veterans Affairs (VA) and The Department of Defense (DoD) guidelines are based on the best information available at the time of publication. They are designed to provide information and assist in decision-making. They are not intended to define a standard of care and should not be construed as one. In addition, they should not be interpreted as prescribing an exclusive course of management.

Variations in practice will inevitably and appropriately occur when providers take into account the needs of individual patients, available resources, and limitations unique to an institution or type of practice. Every healthcare professional making use of these guidelines is responsible for evaluating the appropriateness of applying them in the setting of any particular clinical situation.

Introduction

The Clinical Practice Guideline for the Management of Concussion/Mild Traumatic Brain Injury (mTBI) was developed under the auspices of the Veterans Health Administration (VHA) and the Department of Defense (DoD) pursuant to directives from the Department of Veterans Affairs (VA). VHA and DoD define clinical practice guidelines as:

"Recommendations for the performance or exclusion of specific procedures or services derived through a rigorous methodological approach that includes:

---

* This is an edited, reformatted and augmented version of Department of Veterans Affairs, Department of Defense, dated April, 2009.

- Determination of appropriate criteria such as effectiveness, efficacy, population benefit, or patient satisfaction; and
- Literature review to determine the strength of the evidence in relation to these criteria."

The intent of these guidelines is to:

- Reduce current practice variation and provide facilities with a structured framework to help improve patient outcomes
- Provide evidence-based recommendations to assist providers and their patients in the decision-making process related to the patient health care problems
- Identify outcome measures to support the development of practice-based evidence that can ultimately be used to improve clinical guidelines.

Background

The Centers for Disease Control and Prevention (CDC) has estimated that each year, approximately 1.5 million Americans survive a traumatic brain injury (TBI), among whom approximately 230,000 are hospitalized. Approximately 50,000 Americans die each year following traumatic brain injury, representing one third of all injury-related deaths. The leading causes of TBI are falls (28%), motor vehicle-traffic accidents (20%), struck by/against events (19%) and assaults (11%). It is estimated that of the total reported TBIs, the vast majority (75%-90%) of these fit the categorization of mild-TBI and that approximately ninety percent (90%) of these follow a predictable course and experience few, if any, ongoing symptoms and do not require any special medical treatment. More than 1.1 million patients with mTBI are treated and released from an emergency department each year. Only a small sub-set of these patients (10%) experience post-injury symptoms of a long lasting nature.

The incidence of TBI has significantly increased in the patient population of the DoD and VHA as a result of injuries during recent military and combat operations. In the past 8 years, TBI has emerged as a common form of injury in service men and women serving in Operation Enduring Freedom (OEF) and Operation Iraqi Freedom (OIF). Although penetrating TBI is typically identified and cared for immediately, mTBI may be missed, particularly in the presence of other more obvious injuries. Due to numerous deployments and the nature of enemy tactics, troops are at risk for sustaining more than one mild brain injury or concussion in a short timeframe.

As experience with this condition in OEF and OIF service persons and veterans accumulated, it became clear that screening for possible TBI in OEF and OIF veterans could contribute to ensuring that patients are identified and treatment implemented.

In response to this need, VHA established a task force including members with expertise in Physical Medicine and Rehabilitation, Neurology, Psychiatry, Psychology, Primary Care, Prevention, and Medical Informatics to develop a screening tool and evaluation protocol. Although TBI is a significant public health problem, currently there are no validated screening instruments specific to TBI that are accepted for use in clinical practice. Therefore, the task force reviewed existing literature on screening for TBI, examined the efforts of individual military Medical Treatment Facilities (MTF's) and Department of Veterans Affairs (VA) Medical Centers that had implemented TBI screening locally, consulted with the Defense and Veterans Brain Injury Center (DVBIC), and considered data on the natural history of TBI. Based on these efforts, the task force developed a consensus document that included definitions, classification and taxonomy.

Following the development of a definition document, the task force constructed a screening instrument to assist in identifying OEF and OIF veterans who may be suffering from TBI, and a protocol for further evaluation and treatment of those whose screening tests are positive. Furthermore, a national electronic clinical reminder, VATBI Screening, was built incorporating this screening instrument. These protocols have been considered the seed for the development of this Evidence Based Practice Guideline. The DoD has published Clinical Guidance for Management of Mild-TBI in Theater and mTBI in Non-Deployed Medical Activities.

After the VA/DoD Working Group completed the review of the evidence for this guideline an Institute of Medicine (IOM) report addressing long-term consequences of Traumatic Brain Injury was published (IOM, 2009).

The IOM committee concluded, on the basis of its evaluation, that there is limited/suggestive evidence of an association between sustaining a mild TBI resulting in loss of consciousness or amnesia and the development of unprovoked seizures, ocular and visual motor deterioration.

The committee found inadequate/insufficient evidence to determine whether an association exists between mild TBI and neurocognitive deficits and long-term adverse social functioning, including unemployment, diminished social relationships, and decrease in the ability to live independently.

For long-term outcomes, the IOM report describes limited/suggestive evidence of an association between mild TBI and Parkinson Disorder and between mild TBI and dementia of the Alzheimer's type when the injury included loss of consciousness.

However, insufficient evidence of such association was found in mild TBI without loss of consciousness.

Scope of Guideline

- This Evidence Based Guideline applies to adult patients (18 years or older) who are diagnosed with concussion/mTBI and complain of symptoms related to the injury and who are treated in VA/DoD clinical settings for these symptoms at least 7 days after the initial head injury.
- The guideline is relevant to all healthcare professionals providing or directing treatment services to patients with concussion/mTBI in any VA/DoD healthcare setting, including both primary and specialty care.
- This guideline does not address: management of concussion/mTBI in the acute phase (< 7 days post injury), management of moderate or severe TBI, mTBI presented as polytrauma and managed in an inpatient setting, or mTBI in children

Development Process

The development process of this guideline follows a systematic approach described in "Guideline-forGuidelines," an internal working document of VHA's National Clinical Practice Guideline Counsel.

The literature search identified publications from 2002 through 2008 that addressed adult patients with mTBI. The initial year (2002) was elected to succeed the World Health Organization, (WHO) systematic review of publications related to mTBI conducted in 2002. The WHO Collaborating Centre for Neurotrauma Task Force on Mild Traumatic Brain Injury (Carroll, et al., 2004) performed a comprehensive search and critical review of the literature published between 1980 and 2002 to assemble the best evidence on the epidemiology, diagnosis, prognosis and treatment of mild traumatic brain injury.

The literature identified by the search was critically analyzed and graded using a standardized format applying the evidence grading system used by the U.S. Preventative Services Task Force. For recommendations that are based on evidence the strength of recommendation grade (SR) is included in brackets following the recommendations. Where existing literature was ambiguous or conflicting, or where scientific data were lacking on an issue, recommendations were based on the clinical experience of the members of the Working Group and are presented without an SR grade.

Appendix A fully describes the guideline development process. (See Appendix A – Development Process.)

This Guideline is the product of many months of diligent effort and consensus building among knowledgeable individuals from the VA, DoD, and experts from the private sector. An experienced moderator facilitated the multidisciplinary Working Group.

Implementation

The guideline and algorithms are designed to be adapted to individual facility needs and resources. The algorithms serve as a guide that providers can use to determine best interventions and timing of services for their patients to optimize quality of care and clinical outcomes. This should not prevent providers from using their own clinical expertise in the care of an individual patient. Guideline recommendations are intended to support clinical decision-making but should never replace sound clinical judgment. Although this guideline represents the state of the art practice at the time of its publication, medical practice is evolving and this evolution will require continuous updating of published information. New technologies and increased ongoing research will improve patient care in the future. This clinical practice guideline can assist in identifying priority areas for research and optimal allocation of resources as regards to TBI in general and mTBI in particular. Future studies examining the results of clinical practice guidelines such as these may lead to the development of new practice-based evidence and treatment modalities. A recently developed program that has been created for post-deployment personnel and veterans experiencing head injury deserves mention here. The program for post-deployment care which features an interdisciplinary team of a primary care staff, mental health clinician, and clinical social worker assist in implementation of post-deployment care models across the VA. The providers in these settings have received specialty training in this condition and treatment approaches. Assessment and treatment is organized in a collaborative team model. All referred patients are screened for the need for case management services and all severely ill or injured OIF and OEF patients are case managed.

The Concussion/MTBI Guieline Working Group

VA	DoD
David Cifu, MD	**Amy Bowles, MD**
Robin Hurley, MD	**Douglas Cooper, PhD**
Michelle Peterson, DPT, NCS	**Angela Drake, PhD**
Micaela Cornis-Pop, PhD, SLP	Charles Engel, MD, MPH, COL, USA, MC
Robert L. Ruff, MD, PhD	Lori Simmers Geckle
Patricia A. Rikli, PhD, MSN	**Kathy Helmick, MS, CNRN, CRNP**
Steven G. Scott, DO	Charles Hoge, MD, COL, USA, MC
Kristin A. Silva, RNC, MN, NP	Michael Jaffee, MD, COL, FS, USAF
Barbara J. Sigford, MD, PhD	**Robert Labutta, MD, COL, USA, MC**
Aaron Schneiderman, PhD, MPH, RN	**Geoffrey Ling, MD, PhD, COL, USA, MC**
Gretchen C. Stephens, MPA, OTR/L	Lynne Lowe, PT, DPT, OCS, LTC
Kathryn Tortorice, Pharm D, BCPS	Sheryl Mims, RN
Rodney D. Vanderploeg, PhD, ABPP-CN	Lisa Newman, ScD
Warren Withlock, MD	**David T. Orman, MD, DAC COL**
	Benjamin E. Solomon, MD LTC, USA, MC
	Jay M. Stone, PhD Lt Col, USAF
PRIVATE SECTOR	**Heidi P. Terrio, MD, MPH COL, USA MC**
Jeffrey Barth PhD, ABPP-CN	Kimialeesha Thomas, RN, MSN
Kathleen R. Bell, MD	Mary Tolbert, PA-C
	Christopher S. Williams, MD, COL, USAF
OFFICE OF QUALITY AND PERFORMANCE	**QUALITY MANAGEMENT DIVISION US ARMY MEDICAL COMMAND**
Carla Cassidy, RN, MSN, NP	Ernest Degenhardt, RN, MSN, ANP-FNP, COL, AN
	Angela Klar, RN, MSN, ANP-CS
	Mary Ramos, RN, PhD
FACILITATOR: Oded Susskind, MPH	
RESEARCH: Jessica Cohen, M.S., M.P.H. Jennifer J. Kasten, Ph.D. Sue Radcliff William E. Schlenger, Ph.D.	**HEALTHCARE QUALITY INFORMATICS, INC.** **Martha D'Erasmo, MPH** **Rosalie Fishman, RN, MSN, CPHQ** **Joanne Marko, MS, SLP**

* Bolded names are members of the CORE Editorial Panel.
The complete list of participants and contact information is included in Appendix H.

Future Research

There are unique circumstances related to research of concussion/mTBI that create challenges as regards the development of strong evidence based studies on which to build recommendations and difficulties in determining best practice diagnostic approaches and treatment modalities. These circumstances include: the lack of a standardized definition of mTBI; the fact that much of the literature that does exist is sports-injury based and may not extrapolate successfully to other populations; the fact that the symptoms these patients often exhibit are common to other conditions and that they occur frequently in the population as a whole; the confounding factors related to the existence of pre-morbid or co-occurring diseases or conditions along with the concussion/mTBI; the reality that patients who have suffered a head injury often do not present for treatment for days, weeks, or even months following the initial injury; and the special circumstances surrounding service personnel receiving head injuries in-theatre. **Currently, diagnosis of concussion/mTBI is based primarily on the characteristics of the injury event and not by the severity of symptoms at random points after the trauma.** In addition to the diagnostic difficulties caused by diffuse symptoms of a non-specific nature, the common occurrence of a long time span between injury and presentation for treatment, and the confounding variables of pre-morbid and /or co-occurring morbidities; methodological weaknesses in the literature regarding mTBI are substantial. The World Health Organization (WHO) in its systematic review of the mTBI literature found:

- Differing inception periods, diverse source populations, differing inclusion/exclusion criteria and varying case definitions
- No universally accepted definition of mTBI
- Criteria used by various authors was susceptible to information bias (i.e. using ICD coding to determine) and misclassification of cases
- Many studies did not identify the population at risk that should form the denominator in any incidence calculation.

Successful future research efforts will need to address these methodological difficulties and focus on areas of concern regarding the diagnosis and treatment of concussion/mTBI. For example, many aspects of concussion/mTBI (as with all blunt brain injury) remain confusing, particularly with regards to the spectrum of clinical outcomes that may result. The role of neuropsychological and physiological testing, in an attempt to further characterize the injury, needs additional application and study. The common occurrence of mTBI lends itself to meaningful analysis, both within an institution and in the multi-institutional setting. Enhanced characterization of the mTBI injury will allow more appropriate utilization of the many subspecialists involved in post-traumatic care, including the trauma surgeon; neurologist; physiatrist; physical, cognitive and occupational therapists; psychiatrists; and primary care physicians.

Goals of This Guideline

- To promote evidence-based management of patients diagnosed with mild traumatic brain injury (mTBI)
- To promote efficient and effective assessment of patient's complaints
- To identify the critical decision points in management of patients with concussion/mTBI
- To improve local management of patients with concussion/mTBI and thereby improve patient outcomes
- To promote evidence-based management of individuals with (post-deployment) health concerns related to head injury, blast, or concussion
- To accommodate local policies or procedures, such as those regarding referrals to, or consultation with, specialists

- To motivate administrators at each of the Federal agencies and care access sites to develop innovative plans to break down barriers that may prevent patients from having prompt access to appropriate care
- To diagnose concussion/mTBI accurately and in a timely manner
- To appropriately assess and identify those patients who present with symptoms following a concussion/mTBI or other consequences of head injury
- To identify those patients who may benefit from further assessment, brief intervention and/or ongoing treatment
- To improve the quality and continuum of care for patients with concussion/mTBI
- To identify those patients who may benefit from early intervention and treatment to prevent future complications from concussion/mTBI
- To improve health related outcomes for patients with concussion/mTBI
- To reduce morbidity and mortality from concussion/mTBI.

Document Presentation

- The Guideline is organized around three separate Algorithms:
  - **Algorithm A: Initial Presentation**
  - **Algorithm B: Management of Symptoms**
  - **Algorithm C: Follow-up of Persistent Symptoms**
- Annotations and recommendations in the text match the Box numbers and Letters in the respective algorithms.

  There are a limited number of recommendations that are based on best evidence literature. Therefore, in annotations for which there are evidence based studies to support the recommendations a section titled Evidence Statements follows the recommendations and provides a brief discussion of findings. The Strength of Recommendation [SR] based on the level of evidence is presented in brackets for these recommendations. In annotations for which there is not a body of evidence based literature there is a Discussion Section which discusses approaches defined through assessing expert opinion on the given topic. No SR is presented for these recommendations.

Evidence Rating

A	A strong recommendation that the clinicians provide the intervention to eligible patients. *Good evidence was found that the intervention improves important health outcomes and concludes that benefits substantially outweigh harm.*
B	A recommendation that clinicians provide (the service) to eligible patients. *At least fair evidence was found that the intervention improves health outcomes and concludes that benefits outweigh harm.*
C	No recommendation for or against the routine provision of the intervention is made. *At least fair evidence was found that the intervention can improve health outcomes, but concludes that the balance of benefits and harms is too close to justify a general recommendation.*
D	Recommendation is made against routinely providing the intervention to patients. *At least fair evidence was found that the intervention is ineffective or that harms outweigh benefits.*
I	The conclusion is that the evidence is insufficient to recommend for or against routinely providing the intervention. *Evidence that the intervention is effective is lacking, or poor quality, or conflicting, and the balance of benefits and harms cannot be determined.*

Conventions Used in This Guideline

The terms *concussion* and *mTBI* are used interchangeably. The use of the term concussion or history of mild TBI may be preferred when communicating with the patient, indicating a transient condition, avoiding the use of the terms "brain damage" or "brain injury" that may inadvertently reinforce misperceptions of symptoms or insecurities about recovery. The term *concussion/mTBI* will be used throughout this document as a convention. Two terms commonly used in the literature, Post Concussive Syndrome (PCS) and Post-Concussion Disorder (PCD), also have the potential to reinforce illness behavior and the constellations of symptoms are not accurately described as either a syndrome or disorder. The term Persistent Post-Concussive Symptoms (PPCS) will be used throughout this document as a convention when referring to symptoms related to mTBI that do not remit despite initial treatment.

GUIDELINE KEY POINTS

General

- The management of patients who present with symptoms following a concussion/mTBI injury should focus on promoting recovery and avoiding harm
- A patient-centered approach should be used to provide the needed reassurance and motivation, since patients with prolonged symptoms are suffering, distressed, and in need of guidance, education, support, and understanding
- Currently, there are no universal standard criteria for the definition of concussion/mTBI and the diagnosis is based primarily on the characteristics of the immediate sequelae following the event
- Concussion/mTBI is a common injury, with a time-limited and predictable course. The majority of patients with concussion/mTBI do not require any specific medical treatment
- Experience in contemporary military operations suggests that substantial short-term and long-term neurologic deficits (similar to those following concussion/mTBI) can be caused by blast exposure without a direct blow to the head and may manifested in isolation or part of polytrauma.

Natural Course of Disease

- The vast majority of patients who have sustained a concussion/mTBI improve with no lasting clinical sequelae
- Patients should be reassured and encouraged that the condition is transient and full recovery is expected. The term 'brain damage' should be avoided. A risk communication approach should be applied

- The vast majority of patients recover within hours to days, with a small proportion taking longer. In an even smaller minority, symptoms may persist beyond six months to a year
- The symptoms associated with Post-Concussion Syndrome (PCS) are not unique to mTBI. The symptoms occur frequently in day to day life among healthy individuals and are also found often in persons with other conditions such as chronic pain or depression.

Return to Work /Duty Activity

- Patients sustaining a concussion/mTBI should return to normal (work/duty/school/ leisure) activity post-injury as soon as possible
- A gradual resumption of activity is recommended
- If physical, cognitive, or behavioral complaints/symptoms re-emerge after returning to previous normal activity levels, a monitored progressive return to normal activity as tolerated should be recommended.

Early intervention

- Early education of patients and their families is the best available treatment for concussion/mTBI and for preventing/reducing the development of persistent symptoms
- A primary care model can be appropriate for the management of Concussion/mTBI when implemented by an interdisciplinary team with special expertise.

Symptom Management

- Treatment of somatic complaints (e.g. sleep, dizziness/coordination problems, nausea, numbness, smell/taste, vision, hearing, fatigue, appetite problems) should be based upon individual factors and symptom presentation
- Headache is the single most common symptom associated with concussion/mTBI and assessment and management of headaches in individuals should parallel those for other causes of headache
- Medication for ameliorating the neurocognitive effects attributed to concussion/ mTBI is not recommended
- Medications for headaches, musculoskeletal pain, or depression/anxiety must be carefully prescribed to avoid the sedating properties, which can have an impact upon a person's attention, cognition, and motor performance
- Treatment of psychiatric symptoms following concussion/mTBI should be based upon individual factors and the nature and severity of symptom presentation, and may include both psychotherapeutic and pharmacological treatment modalities

- In patients with persistent post-concussive symptoms (PPCS), which have been refractory to treatment, consideration should be given to other factors including psychiatric, psychosocial support, and compensatory/litigation.

ALGORITHMS

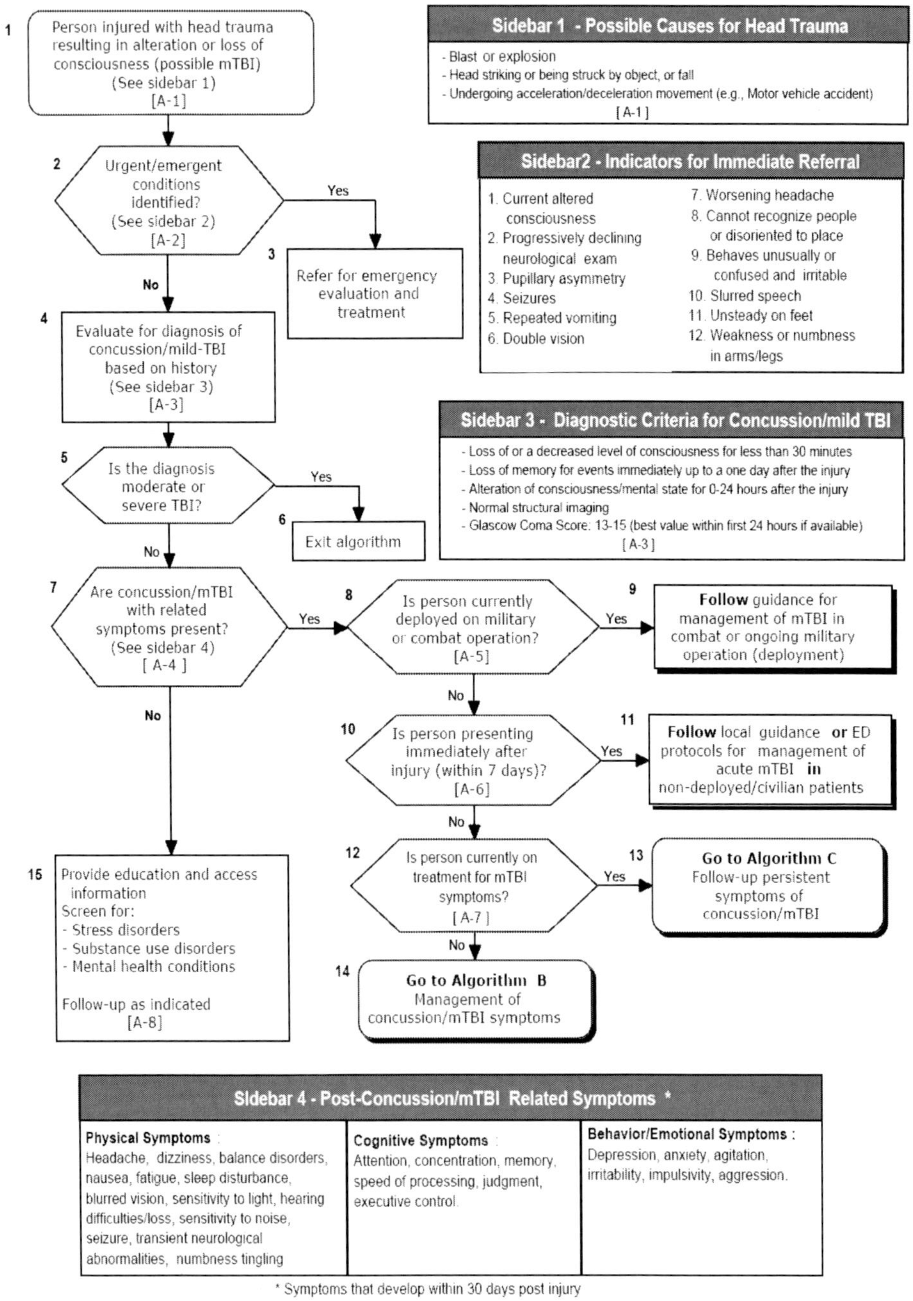

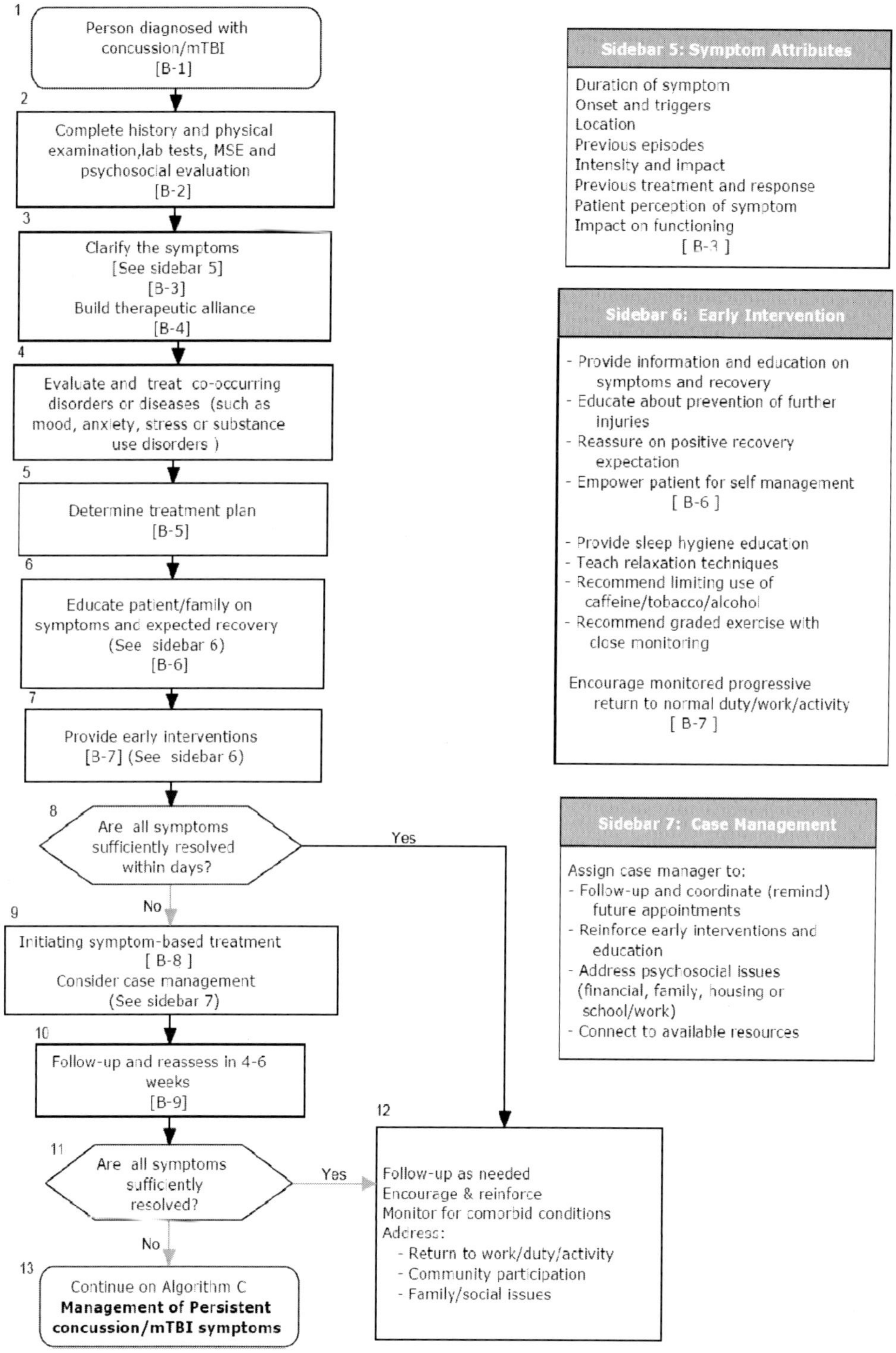
1
Person diagnosed with concussion/mTBI [B-1]
2
Complete history and physical examination,lab tests, MSE and psychosocial evaluation [B-2]
3
Clarify the symptoms [See sidebar 5] [B-3] Build therapeutic alliance [B-4]
4
Evaluate and treat co-occurring disorders or diseases (such as mood, anxiety, stress or substance use disorders)
5
Determine treatment plan [B-5]
6
Educate patient/family on symptoms and expected recovery (See sidebar 6) [B-6]
7
Provide early interventions [B-7] (See sidebar 6)
8
Are all symptoms sufficiently resolved within days?
Yes
No
9
Initiating symptom-based treatment [B-8] Consider case management (See sidebar 7)
10
Follow-up and reassess in 4-6 weeks [B-9]
11
Are all symptoms sufficiently resolved?
Yes
No
12
Follow-up as needed
Encourage & reinforce
Monitor for comorbid conditions
Address:
- Return to work/duty/activity
- Community participation
- Family/social issues
13
Continue on Algorithm C
Management of Persistent concussion/mTBI symptoms
Sidebar 5: Symptom Attributes
Duration of symptom
Onset and triggers
Location
Previous episodes
Intensity and impact
Previous treatment and response
Patient perception of symptom
Impact on functioning
[B-3]
Sidebar 6: Early Intervention
- Provide information and education on symptoms and recovery
- Educate about prevention of further injuries
- Reassure on positive recovery expectation
- Empower patient for self management
[B-6]
- Provide sleep hygiene education
- Teach relaxation techniques
- Recommend limiting use of caffeine/tobacco/alcohol
- Recommend graded exercise with close monitoring
Encourage monitored progressive return to normal duty/work/activity
[B-7]
Sidebar 7: Case Management
Assign case manager to:
- Follow-up and coordinate (remind) future appointments
- Reinforce early interventions and education
- Address psychosocial issues (financial, family, housing or school/work)
- Connect to available resources

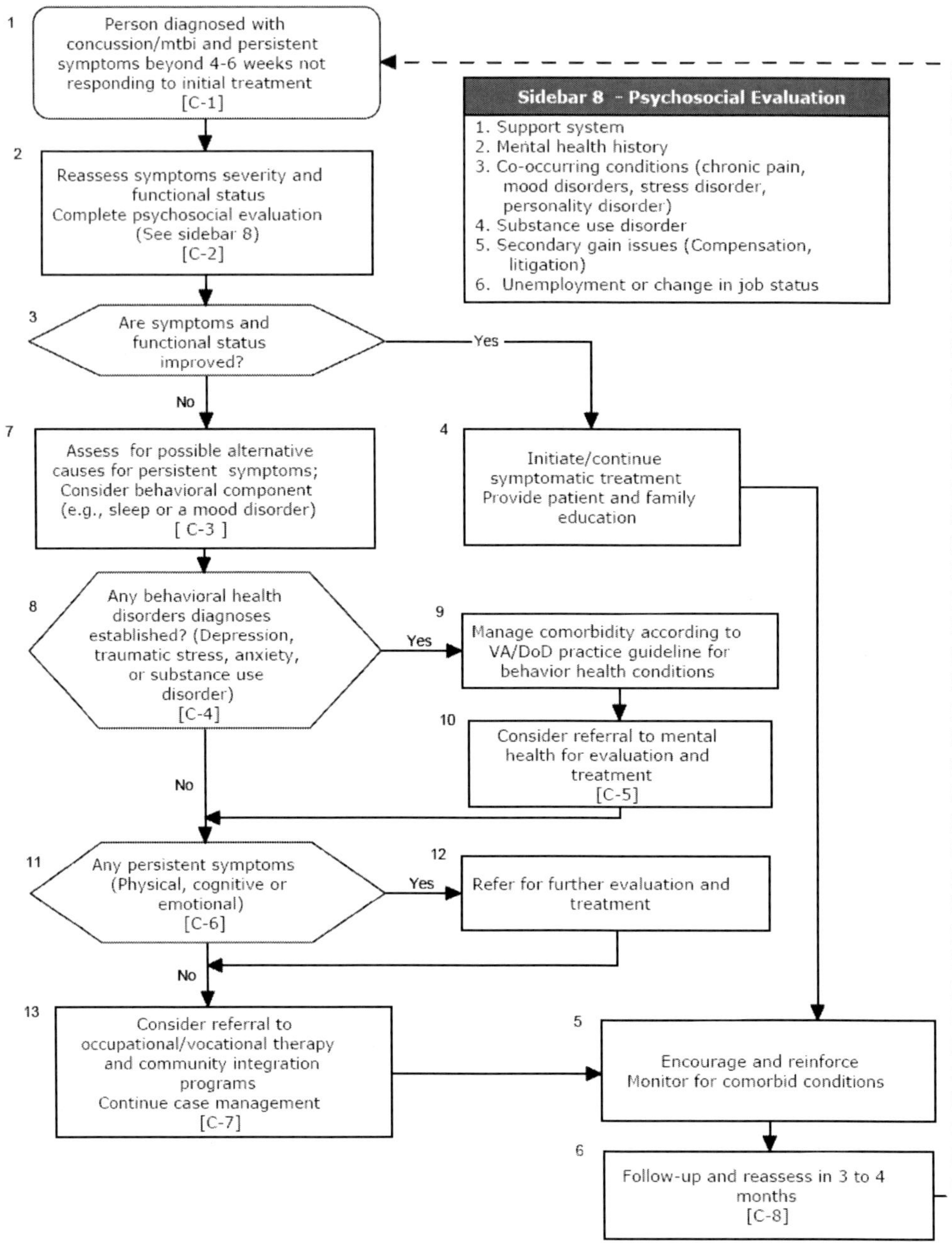

A: Initial Presentation

Annotation A-1 Person Injured with Head Trauma Resulting in Possible Alteration or Loss of Consciousness

1. Definitions/Classifications

1.1. Definition of Traumatic Brain Injury

A traumatically induced structural injury and/or physiological disruption of brain function as a result of an external force that is indicated by new onset or worsening of at least one of the following clinical signs, immediately following the event:

- Any period of loss of or a decreased level of consciousness (LOC)
- Any loss of memory for events immediately before or after the injury (post-traumatic amnesia [PTA])
- Any alteration in mental state at the time of the injury (confusion, disorientation, slowed thinking, etc.) (Alteration of consciousness /mental state [AOC])
- Neurological deficits (weakness, loss of balance, change in vision, praxis, paresis/plegia, sensory loss, aphasia, etc.) that may or may not be transient
- Intracranial lesion.

External forces may include any of the following events: the head being struck by an object, the head striking an object, the brain undergoing an acceleration/deceleration movement without direct external trauma to the head, a foreign body penetrating the brain, forces generated from events such as a blast or explosion, or other forces yet to be defined.

The above criteria define the event of a TBI. Not all individuals exposed to an external force will sustain a TBI, but any person who has a history of such an event with immediate manifestation of any of the above signs and symptoms can be said to have had a TBI.

1.2. Severity of Brain Injury Stratification

TBI is further categorized as to severity into mild, moderate, or severe based on the length of LOC, AOC, or PTA (see Table A-1). Acute injury severity is determined at the time of the injury.

- The patient is classified as mild/moderate/severe if s/he meets any of the criteria in Table A-1 within a particular severity level. If a patient meets criteria in more than one category of severity, the higher severity level is assigned.
- If it is not clinically possible to determine the brain injury level of severity because of medical complications (e.g., medically induced coma), other severity markers are required to make a determination of the severity of the brain injury.
- Abnormal structural imaging (e.g., Magnetic Resonance Imaging or Computed Tomography Scanning) attributed to the injury will result in the individual being considered clinically to have greater than mild injury.

In addition to traditional imaging studies, other imaging techniques such as functional magnetic resonance imaging, diffusion tensor imaging, positron emission tomography scanning; electrophysiological testing such as electroencephalography; and neuropsychological or other standardized testing of function have been used in the evaluation of persons with TBIs, but are not considered in the currently accepted criteria for measuring severity at the time of the acute injury outlined in Table A-1.

The severity level has prognostic value, but does not necessarily predict the patient's ultimate level of functioning. There is substantial evidence that the epidemiology, pathophysiology, natural history, and prognosis for concussion/mTBI are different than for moderate and severe TBI.

For example, moderate and severe TBI are often associated with objective evidence of brain injury on brain scan or neurological examination (e.g., neurological deficits) and objective deficits on neuropsychological testing, whereas these evaluations are frequently not definitive in persons with concussion/mTBI.

The natural history and prognosis of moderate and severe TBI are much more directly related to the nature and severity of the injury in moderate and severe TBI, whereas factors unrelated to the injury (such as co-existing mental disorders) have been shown to be the strong predictors of symptom persistence after a concussion/mTBI.

Concussion: The terms *concussion* and *mTBI* can be used interchangeably. The use of the term concussion or history of mild TBI may be preferred when communicating with the patient, indicating a transient condition, avoiding the use of the terms "brain damage" or "brain injury" that may inadvertently reinforce misperceptions of symptoms or insecurities about recovery. The patient who is told s/he has "brain damage" based on vague symptoms complaints and no clear indication of significant head trauma may develop a long-term perception of disability that is difficult to undo (Wood, 2004).

The term *concussion/mTBI* will be used throughout this document as a convention.

Table A-1. Classification of TBI Severity

Criteria	Mild	Moderate	Severe
Structural imaging	Normal	Normal or abnormal	Normal or abnormal
Loss of Consciousness (LOC)	0–30 min	> 30 min and < 24 hrs	> 24 hrs
Alteration of consciousness/mental state (AOC) *	a moment up to 24 hrs	> 24 hours. Severity based on other criteria	
Post-traumatic amnesia (PTA)	0–1 day	> 1 and < 7 days	> 7 days
Glascow Coma Scale (best available score in first 24 hours)	13-15	9-12	< 9

* Alteration of mental status must be immediately related to the trauma to the head. Typical symptoms would be: looking and feeling dazed and uncertain of what is happening, confusion, difficulty thinking clearly or responding appropriately to mental status questions, and being unable to describe events immediately before or after the trauma event.

Annotation A-2 *Urgent/emergent conditions identified?*

Recommendations: 1. The following physical findings, signs and symptoms ("Red Flags") may indicate an acute neurologic condition that requires urgent specialty consultation (neurology, neuro-surgical) :

a.	Altered consciousness	h.	Cannot recognize people or is disoriented to place
c.	Pupillary asymmetry	i.	Behaves unusually or seems confused and irritable
d.	Seizures	j.	Slurred speech
e.	Repeated vomiting	k.	Unsteady on feet
f.	Double vision	l.	Weakness or numbness in arms / legs
g.	Worsening headache		

Annotation A-3 Evaluate for Diagnosis of Concussion/mTBI, Based on History

1.3. Diagnostic Criteria for mTBI

Background: In the U.S., the most widely accepted criteria for mild TBI are those proposed by the American College of Rehabilitation Medicine (ACRM, 1993). They are "a physiological disruption of brain function as a result of a traumatic event as manifested by at least one of the following: alteration of mental state, loss of consciousness (LOC), loss of memory or focal neurological deficit, that may or may not be transient; but where the severity of the injury does not exceed the following: post-traumatic amnesia (PTA) for greater than 24 hours, after the first 30 minutes Glasgow Coma Score (GCS) 13 - 15, and loss of consciousness is less than 30 minutes." There are other criteria used by other medical groups. However, most agree that common criteria include GCS score of 13-15, brief LOC, brief PTA and negative head computed tomography (CT) scan.

Recommendations: 1. A diagnosis of mTBI should be made when there is an injury to the head as a result of blunt trauma, acceleration or deceleration forces or exposure to blast that result in one or more of the following conditions:

a. Any period of observed or self-reported:

- Transient confusion, disorientation, or impaired consciousness
- Dysfunction of memory immediately before or after the time of injury
- Loss of consciousness (LOC) lasting less than 30 minutes.

b. Observed signs of neurological or neuropsychological dysfunction, such as:

- Headache, dizziness, irritability, fatigue or poor concentration, when identified soon after injury, can be used to support the diagnosis of mild TBI, but cannot be used to make the diagnosis in the absence of loss of consciousness or altered consciousness.

2. The severity of TBI must be defined by the acute injury characteristics and not by the severity of symptoms at random points after trauma.

Discussion: The lack of standardized criteria and the variable quality of the current literature on mTBI (Carroll et al., 2004), poses the risk of misclassification of patients with concussion symptoms. Although this is an important issue for research, the implications for care could cause over- or under-diagnosing of patients with mTBI. This led the Working Group to rely on expert opinion in determining recommendations for intervention.

Annotation A-4 Are Concussion/mTBI with Related Symptoms Present

1.4. Symptoms Associated with Concussion/mTBI

Concussion/mTBI is associated with a variety of symptoms that will manifest immediately following the event, and may resolve quickly, within minutes to hours after the injury event, or they may persist longer. The most typical signs and symptoms after concussion fall into one or more of the following three categories:

a) Physical: headache, nausea, vomiting, dizziness, fatigue, blurred vision, sleep disturbance, sensitivity to light/noise, balance problems, transient neurological abnormalities
b) Cognitive: attention, concentration, memory, speed of processing, judgment, executive function
c) Behavioral/emotional: depression, anxiety, agitation, irritability, impulsivity, aggression.

Signs and symptoms may occur alone or in varying combinations and may result in functional impairment.

Although a variety of symptoms can occur in association with TBI, they are *not* part of the definition of TBI, and there are no pathognomonic symptoms or signs. The term "mild TBI" refers only to the initial injury severity and should not be interpreted referring to the level of the severity of the symptoms.

Signs and symptoms, following the concussion, should not be attributed to concussion/mTBI if they are better explained by pre-existing conditions or other medical, neurological, or psychological causes except in cases of an immediate exacerbation of a pre-existing condition.

Symptoms associated with concussion/mTBI are not unique. These symptoms occur frequently in day-to-day life among healthy individuals and are often found in persons with other conditions such as chronic pain, depression or other traumatic injuries. These symptoms are also common to any number of preexisting/pre-morbid conditions the patient may have had.

Each patient tends to exhibit a different mix of symptoms and the symptoms themselves are highly subjective in nature. Research studies do not offer strong support for a consistent pattern of the types of symptoms occurrence and resolution following mild TBI. Symptoms do not appear to cluster together in a uniform, or even in a consistent expected trend. The presence of somatic symptoms is not linked predictably to the presence of neuropsychiatric (i.e., cognitive, emotional, or behavioral) symptoms, and the neuropsychiatric consequences of mTBI are not linked consistently to one another. Additionally, there is little evidence of coupling of symptom resolution following mTBI. Few persons with multiple post-concussion symptoms experience persistence of the entire set of their symptoms over time. (Arciniegas, 2005)

This lack of symptom consistency may reflect the complex effects of head injury on the brain and also the interaction between the injury and each individual's pre- or post-injury psychosocial factors (Alexander 1995; King 1996).

Annotation A-5 Is Person Currently Deployed on Combat or Ongoing Military Operation?

Recommendations: 1. Management of service members presenting for care immediately after a head injury (within 7 days) during military combat or ongoing operation should follow guidelines for acute management published by DoD. (See: Recommendations for acute management of concussion/mTBI in the deployed setting, Defense and Veterans Brain Injury Center Consensus August, 2008)

(This guidance is not included in this evidence-based guideline.)

Annotation A-6 Is Person Presenting Immediately (Within 7 Days) After Injury? (Non-Military/Civilian Setting)

Recommendations: 1. Management of non-deployed service members, veterans, or civilian patients presenting for care immediately after a head injury (within 7 days) should follow guidelines for acute management. (See Recommendations for acute management in guideline published by the American College of Emergency Medicine and the Center for Disease Control and Prevention (ACEP/CDC, 2008)

(These protocols and guidance are not included in this evidence-based guideline.)

1.5. Post Deployment Delayed Awareness and Delayed Reporting of Symptoms

Background: The elapsed time since the exposure to the head injury (trauma) and the self-reporting of symptoms by the patient to their primary care provider may vary. This period is very important in assessing the risk of developing concussion/mTBI symptoms and determining the appropriate intervention.

The concussion/mTBI algorithms are designed to accommodate patients entering the healthcare system at different intervals post-injury. Algorithm A (Initial Presentation) describes a new entry into the healthcare system and is not dependent on the time since injury. It does not follow the traditional acute, sub-acute, and post-acute phases of brain injury. This is particularly important with combat-related TBI that may inherently lead to delays in seeking treatment due to discounting or misattributing symptoms, and reluctance to report health problems. The initial management of symptoms related to concussion/mTBI is then described in Algorithm B (Management of Symptoms). Algorithm C (Follow-up Persistent Symptoms) will apply to any service person/veteran for whom treatment of concussion symptoms previously had been started.

1.5.1. Initial Stages following mTBI/Concussion

Example: Individual sustains a head injury and presents to a provider two weeks following the injury. The provider uses Algorithm A to diagnose concussion/mTBI, and Algorithm B to initiate the management of symptoms. If the symptoms do not remit within 4 to 6 weeks of the initial treatment, the provider follows Algorithm C to manage the persistent symptoms.

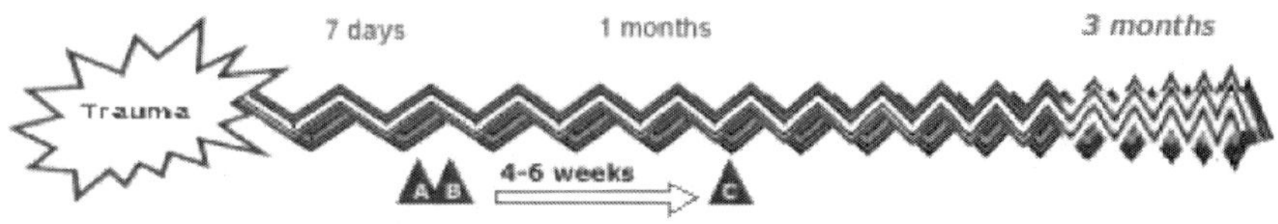

Figure 1. Initial Stages following mTBI/Concussion.

1.5.2. Delayed Initial Presentation of Symptoms

Example: Individual sustains a head injury followed by experiencing of symptoms. The patient does not access medical care for weeks or months post-injury. Despite the long elapsed time since injury, the provider uses Algorithm A and B for the initial work-up to make the diagnosis and initiate treatment. This initial treatment may be provided in a setting designated for diagnosis and management of mTBI. If the symptoms do not remit within 4 to 6 weeks of the initial treatment, the provider follows Algorithm C to manage the persistent symptoms.

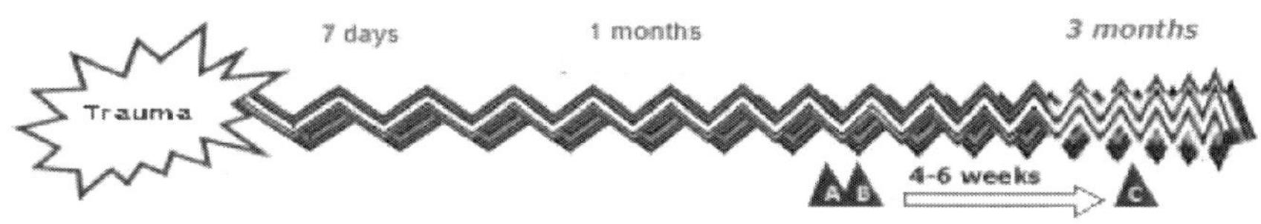

Figure 1. Delayed Initial Presentation of Symptoms.

Recommendations:

1) Service members or veterans identified by post deployment screening or who present with symptoms should be assessed and diagnosed according to ***Algorithm A – Initial Presentation***. The initial evaluation and management will then follow the recommendations in ***Algorithm B*** – Management ***of Symptoms***.
2) Patients who continue to complain of concussion/mTBI-related symptoms beyond 4 to 6 weeks after treatment has been initiated, should have the assessment for these chronic symptoms repeated and should be managed using ***Algorithm C – Follow-up Persistent Symptoms.***
3) Patients who continue to have persistent symptoms despite treatment for persistent symptoms (Algorithm C) beyond 2 years post-injury do not require repeated assessment for these chronic symptoms and should be conservatively managed using a simple symptom-based approach.
4) Patients with symptoms that develop more than 30 days after a concussion should have a focused diagnostic work-up specific to those symptoms only. These symptoms are highly unlikely to be the result of the concussion and therefore the work-up and management should not focus on the initial concussion.

Discussion: Posttraumatic complaints after concussion/mTBI are not well understood. This ambiguity can be further attributed to: issues associated with delays in seeking treatment; providers' lack of knowledge about the detection and diagnosis of mTBI (CDC, 2003); symptom overlap with other diagnoses or conditions (Borg et al., 2004); patients seeking benefit from litigation claims (Binder & Rohling, 1996) or an underlying mood disorder (Rapoport et al., 2003). Unfortunately, there are no sensitive diagnostic tools or biochemical markers that correlate uniquely to concussion/mTBI symptom reports (Borg et al., 2004).

Several authors advocate use of standard criteria for defining mTBI. Indeed, in a review article, Kushner (1998) suggests that mild TBI can be misleading as a diagnostic term as it may include a spectrum of manifestations ranging from transient mild symptoms to ongoing disabling problems.

Symptomatic individuals will frequently present days, weeks, or even months after the trauma. These delays are associated with the injured person discounting symptoms, incorrectly interpreting symptoms, guilt over the circumstances involved in the injury, and denial that anything serious occurred (Mooney et al., 2005). Delay in seeking treatment may be important in mTBI recovery, where reports indicate that early interventions to reduce disability are most effective when provided during the initial post injury phase (McCrea, 2007).

Annotation A-7 *Is Person Currently on Treatment for mTBI Symptoms?*

1.6. Persistent Symptoms after Concussion/mTBI

Background: Most symptoms and signs that occur in the acute period following a single concussion resolve quickly (within hours or days) after the injury. There is debate about the incidence of developing persistent symptoms after concussion, largely due to the lack of an accepted case definition for persistent symptoms and the fact that none of the symptoms are specific to concussion. There is no consensus on a case definition for persistent symptoms attributed to concussion/mTBI and no consensus on the time course when acute symptoms should be considered persistent. As a result, the important focus should be on treating the symptoms rather than on determining the etiology of the symptoms.

Recommendations: Persons who complain about somatic, cognitive or behavioral difficulties after concussion/mTBI should be assessed and treated symptomatically regardless of the elapsed time from injury.

1) The assessment of an individual with persistent concussion /mTBI related symptoms should be directed to the specific nature of the symptoms regardless of their etiology.
2) The management of an individual who has sustained a documented concussion/mTBI and has *persistent* physical, cognitive and behavioral symptoms after one month should not differ based on the specific underlying etiology of their symptoms (i.e., concussion vs. pain, concussion vs. stress disorder).
3) In communication with patients and the public, this guideline recommends using the term *concussion* or *history of mild-TBI* and to refrain from using the term 'brain damage'.

Discussion: It can be difficult to clinically determine if symptoms are attributable to concussion. This difficulty is due to the subjective nature of these symptoms, the very high base rates of many of these symptoms in normal populations (Iverson, 2003; Wang, 2006), and the many other etiologies that can be associated with these symptoms. Common conditions that may present with similar symptoms include PTSD, depression, anxiety disorders, pain, other injuries, and disorders such as fibromyalgia, medical side-effects, and negative illness perceptions by patients (Iverson et al., 2007).

Since post-concussive symptoms may occur as non-specific responses to trauma, studies compare patients with concussions to patients with other types of trauma. Results are inconsistent. In a cross sectional study of Vietnam veterans with a history of mild TBI compared with a history of other injuries, the prevalence of post-concussive symptoms were significantly higher in the mTBI group (Vanderploeg, 2007). Research has yielded inconsistent evidence about acute neuropsychological differences between patients with mTBI with PCS symptoms and controls (Landre 2006; Ponsford et al., 2000). Several studies have shown that persons with non-head traumas have similar rates of "post-concussion syndrome" or symptoms compared with persons with a concussions/mTBI, both in the acute period and out to 3 months post-injury. Therefore, not only are these symptoms non-specific responses to trauma, it is also unclear if timing of the onset of symptoms can be helpful in determining if they are due to the concussion (Boake et. al., 2005; Landre, 2006; McCauley, 2001; Meares et al., 2008).

Somatic, cognitive, and behavioral symptoms after concussion/mTBI rapidly resolve by 2 to 4 weeks in the majority of individuals (McCrea, 2003). "Post-concussion syndrome" (PCS) is a term frequently used to describe a constellation of symptoms that clinicians have described as occurring at least 1 to 3 months after concussion.

The association of post-concussion syndrome with concussion has not met generally accepted epidemiological criteria for causation. There are two commonly used case definitions, one from the Diagnostic and Statistical Manual for Mental Disorders (DSM-IV-TR, 2000) and the other included in the International Statistical Classification of Diseases and Related Health Problems 10th Revision (ICD-10). A study that directly compared the two definitions showed poor correlation between them and there was no way to determine which one is more accurate (Boake et al., 2004).

Another study indicated that the ICD-10 definition "accurately classified" mTBI patients one month after the concussion injury, but was unable to after 3 months (Kashluba et al., 2000).

Because symptoms of PCS are not specific to mTBI, the use of ICD-10 diagnostic criteria for PCS is problematic and may be misleading as it incorrectly suggests that the basis of PCS is a brain injury (Carroll et al., 2004).

The term post-concussion syndrome (PCS) is used in the literature for individuals who have persistent non-focal, neurologic symptoms (at least two). These are most commonly dizziness, headache, cognitive deficits (attention, memory, and judgment), behavioral changes (irritability, depression, nightmares) and/or sleep disturbance, at between one month (ICD-10, 1992) and three months (DSM-IV definition, 1994) postmTBI. PCS is seen in between 15% (DSM-IV) to 50% (WHO-ICD-10) of persons with mTBI, depending on how it is defined (McCrea, 2003).

Various studies of persisting symptoms have employed various symptom checklists rather than uniform criteria-based diagnoses. As a result, large differences are reported in the frequency of patients meeting the diagnostic criteria sets. Some have argued that the rate of 15percent, initially reported by many, is incorrect and argued that the more accurate rate may be closer to 3-5 percent (Iverson, 2007; McCrea, 2007).

Annotation A-8 Provide Education and Access Information; Follow-Up as Indicated

1.7. Follow-Up and Monitoring

It is important to closely monitor the injured person for concussion/mTBI related symptoms and provide supportive education over the initial 30 days. Individuals who sustain a concussion/mTBI and are asymptomatic can be reassured and advised about precautionary measures to prevent future head injury.

Recommendations:

1) Individuals who sustain a concussion/mTBI and are asymptomatic should be reassured about recovery and advised about precautionary measures to prevent future head injury.
2) Patients should be provided with written contact information and be advised to contact their healthcare provider for follow-up if their condition deteriorates or they develop symptoms.
3) Individuals who sustain a concussion/mTBI and are asymptomatic should be screened for comorbid mental health disorders (MDD, PTSD, and SUD) and dangerousness.

B: Management of Concussion/MTBI Symptoms

Annotation B-1 *Person Diagnosed with Concussion/mTBI*

2. Initial Presentation

The vast majority of individuals with concussion/mTBI will have no difficulties or complaints lasting more than a couple of weeks following the injury.

Although, early interventions have been shown to prevent symptoms, some persons sustaining a concussion/mTBI during deployment will not receive early diagnosis or will not seek treatment, and therefore their symptoms will be addressed only after a temporal delay. This guideline recommends that these individuals will be first treated following the algorithm and annotations in Algorithms A and B. If treatment has already been rendered for concussion/mTBI related symptoms and despite treatment the patient continues to experience symptoms, the management will follow recommendations in Algorithm C.

Patients managed in Algorithm B are service persons or veterans identified by post deployment screening, or who present to care with symptoms or complaints related to head injury.

Patients presenting for care immediately after head injury (within 7 days) should follow guidelines for acute management and should not use this algorithm. (See Annotation A-5 and A-6)

Annotation B-2 *Complete a History, Physical Examination; Minimal Mental Examination and Psychosocial Evaluation*

3. Assessment of Symptoms and Severity

3.1. History, Physical Examination, Laboratory Tests, Imaging

Background: Although the initial part of the screening process for mild TBI depends on self-report, the second-level assessment relies on obtaining a careful detailed medical history, physical examination, and a psychosocial assessment. The goal of the assessment is to evaluate the symptoms in order to optimize care, to improve outcomes, and ultimately reduce disability following a concussion/mTBI. It is recognized that patients may not present for medical care immediately following concussion/mTBI. Therefore, the purpose of the assessment may vary slightly based on the timing of the presentation following injury. For patients presenting immediately after the injury event, assessment will include the necessity to rule out neurosurgical emergencies. In patients who present with delayed injury-to assessment intervals, the assessment will include confirmation linking the symptoms to the concussive event. Regardless of the time that has elapsed since injury, management should begin with the patient's first presentation for treatment.

3.1.1. History

Taking an accurate history is an essential part of the diagnostic work-up. The first and most critical step in the evaluation of persons with possible concussion symptoms should clearly characterize the initial injury and determine whether the symptoms are temporally related to the event characterized as a concussion/mTBI.

Recommendations:

1) Individuals who are presumed to have symptoms related to concussion/mTBI or who are identified as positive for mTBI on the initial screening should receive specific assessment of their symptoms.
2) Medical history should include the following:
   a) Obtaining detailed information on the patient's symptoms and health concerns.
   b) Obtaining detailed information of the injury event including mechanism of injury, duration and severity of alteration of consciousness, immediate symptoms, symptom course and prior treatment
   c) Screening for pre-morbid conditions, potential co-occurring conditions or other psychosocial risk factors, such as substance use disorders that may exacerbate or

maintain current symptom presentation (using standardized screening tools such as, PHQ-2, Audit-C, PTSD screen)

d) Evaluating signs and symptoms indicating potential for neurosurgical emergencies that require immediate referrals

e) Assessing of danger to self or others.

3) Patient's experiences should be validated by allowing adequate time for building a provider-patient alliance and applying a risk communication approach. (See Appendix B: Structured Interview for Collecting Head Trauma Event Characteristics)

Discussion:

- Clarifying pre-injury developmental, medical, neurological, psychiatric, academic, and employment histories are essential, particularly in regards to conditions that may influence recovery following mild TBI.
- Psychiatric and substance disorders, cranial and cervical trauma, and other primary neurological and somatic disorders may produce symptoms that overlap with those commonly produced by TBI.
- Persons sustaining concussion/mTBI are at risk for the harmful and potentially addictive use of alcohol, medication, and illicit drugs. Standardized screening instruments should be used to screen for these conditions. (See VA/DoD clinical practice guidelines for mental health disorders). A concussion is not a contraindication for referral to a substance abuse treatment program.

3.1.2. Physical Examination

Recommendations:

2. The physical examination of the person sustaining a concussion/mTBI should focus on the following:

a) A focused neurologic examination, including a Mental Status Examination (MSE), cranial nerve testing, extremity tone testing, deep tendon reflexes, strength, sensation, and postural stability (Romberg's Test, dynamic standing)

b) A focused vision examination including gross acuity, eye movement, binocular function and visual fields/attention testing

c) A focused musculoskeletal examination of the head and neck, including range of motion of the neck and jaw, and focal tenderness and referred pain.

3. The following physical findings, signs and symptoms ("Red Flags") may indicate an acute neurologic condition that requires urgent specialty consultation (neurology, neuro-surgical):

a) Altered consciousness

b) Progressively declining neurological examination

c) Pupillary asymmetry

d) Seizures

e) Repeated vomiting

f) Double vision

g) Worsening headache

h) Cannot recognize people or is disoriented to place

i) Behaves unusually or seems confused and irritable

j) Slurred speech
k) Unsteady on feet
l) Weakness or numbness in arms/legs.

3.1.3. Laboratory Tests

Background: Because diagnostic and cognitive tests have limited ability to predict long-term outcomes for persons with concussion/mTBI, investigators are focused on searching for biochemical markers that may be useful in diagnosis and prognosis.

Recommendations:

1) Laboratory testing is not necessary to confirm or manage symptoms associated with concussion/mTBI.
2) Laboratory testing may be considered for evaluating other non-TBI causes of the symptoms presented.
3) There is insufficient evidence to support the use of serum biomarkers for concussion/mTBI in clinical practice. [SR = I]

Evidence Statements: *Does research identify biomarkers that may be useful in the diagnosis and prognosis of concussion/mTBI?*

Biomarker research has not identified markers with clinical utility in management of mTBI. The biomarker that has been most widely studied, S-100B, is only detectable in the first few hours after injury. The Working Group reviewed 30 studies that were identified by the search. Only 8 met the inclusion criteria and were utilized in the final analysis.

- Elevated S-100B has been associated with abnormal CT scans (Biberthaler, 2001), and prolonged duration prior to return to work (Stranjalis et al., 2004) but has also been detected in other types of trauma, soft tissue injuries, burns, and in vigorous physical activity (Mussack et al., 2003; Stalnacke et al., 2003).
- At this time, there is no consistent marker that is useful in the acute or post-acute periods for mTBI (Iverson et al., 2007).
- S-100B (corrected or uncorrected) and C-tau have not been shown to be predictive of the development of post-concussive syndrome (Bazarian et al., 2006; Bazarian et al., 2006). In addition, S-100B has not been shown to be related to the development of headaches at three months (Bazarian et al., 2006).
- Immediately following acute concussion/mTBI, a normal S-100B test (i.e., absent) in the absence of clinical findings of nausea, dizziness, neck pain, or vomiting correlates with absence of post-concussive syndrome at six months. (de Krujik et al., 2002).

3.1.4. Imaging

Background: The role of neuroimaging in diagnosing concussion/mTBI continues to evolve and be debated in the literature. Various neuroimaging modalities can be employed in helping to identify structural neuropathology. Structural imaging modalities include Computed Tomography (CT) Scan, Magnetic Resonance Imaging (MRI) Diffusion Tensor

Imaging (DTI). Functional imaging modalities include Single Photon Emission Computed Tomography (SPECT), Positron Emission Tomography (PET) and functional

MRI (fMRI). However, many of these modalities are still at the preliminary/research stage of development. Currently, CT scan is the modality of choice as a diagnostic tool for acute concussion/mTBI. The absence of abnormal findings on CT does not preclude the presence of concussion/mTBI.

Recommendations:

1) A patient who presents with any signs or symptoms that may indicate an acute neurologic condition that requires urgent intervention should be referred for evaluation that may include neuroimaging studies.
2) Neuroimaging is not recommended in patients who sustained a concussion/mTBI beyond the emergency phase (72 hours post-injury) except if the condition deteriorates or red flags are noted.

Discussion: Since neuroimaging studies are not necessary for all patients with concussion/mTBI beyond the acute phase, the Working Group did not review the literature regarding the use of neuroimaging in mTBI.

In general, structural imaging techniques play a role in acute diagnosis and management, while functional imaging techniques are being evaluated in an attempt to clarify the pathophysiology, symptom genesis and mechanism of recovery from concussion/mTBI (McAllister et al., 2001). The primary objective of the initial clinical evaluation of patients sustaining a concussion/mTBI is the immediate detection of any neurological deterioration. In particular, patients who exhibit a declining neurologic status, including progressive lethargy, pupillary dilatation, or focal neurologic deficit not explained by systemic sources, should have an urgent CT scanning and neurosurgical consultation. Patients with signs and symptoms indicating an acute neurologic condition should be referred for urgent evaluation.

After a concussion/mTBI, there is a very small risk of intracranial hematoma. The presence of this potentially fatal complication may become apparent only after there is clinical deterioration. Consequently, a cranial CT may be utilized in the acute evaluation of concussion/mTBI to exclude the possibility of occult hematoma. Other imaging techniques may be used to investigate persistent symptoms and deterioration. The provider requires very clear decision rules for the appropriate use of a CT in the acute evaluation of concussion/mTBI.

3.2. Multiple Concussions

Background: Some patients presenting for an initial evaluation may report a history of repeated concussions that have worsened their symptoms. The approach of symptom-based assessment and treatment of repeated concussion should be similar to the management of exposure to a single injury.

Recommendations:

1) The management of a patient who has sustained multiple concussions should be similar to the management for a single concussion/mTBI. [SR = I]

2) The patient with multiple concussions and his/her family should be educated to create a positive expectation of recovery. [SR = I]

Evidence Statements:

Is there a difference in interventions in individuals with repeated concussion/mTBI?

Out of 17 studies identified by the initial search, 10 studies were included for further review of full text documents. Five of those studies met inclusion criteria for evaluating the effect of multiple concussions.

The evidence is inconsistent regarding whether or not cumulative concussions are associated with worse or longer recovery.

- Most studies are based on self-reported data of historical concussions. As a whole, many studies are difficult to interpret because of potential confounders. Some research tools have demonstrated subtle abnormalities in the presence of normal clinical presentations and neuropsychological test performance. Two well-controlled studies of football concussions reached opposite conclusions regarding the cumulative impact of three or more concussions. The NCAA study (Guskiewicz et al., 2003) showed a dose response relationship in duration of neurocognitive recovery associated with multiple concussions in the acute period after injury, whereas the NFL study (Pellman et al., 2004) showed no such relationship.
- The literature is insufficient to conclude that there is an association between mild TBI and neurodegenerative disorders (e.g., Alzheimers disease) although there is evidence that patients with severe TBIs may have increased risk (Guskiewicz et. al., 2005; Mehta et al., 1999).
- History of prior head injury has been shown to be associated with poorer outcomes in terms of lingering symptoms (Binder, 1997; Ponsford et al., 2000).

Annotation B-3 *Clarify the Symptoms*

3.3. Assessment of Symptoms

Background: Patients who have sustained a concussion/mTBI may complain about post-injury symptoms that can be grouped into three categories: physical, cognitive, and emotional/behavioral. (See Annotation A-4) The clinical presentation is expected to include at least some elements of the classic constellation of post-concussive symptoms and gradual, although sometimes incomplete, symptomatic improvement over time.

Although post-concussive symptoms (PCS) are most often discussed in the context of mTBI, these terms and their clinical referents are not synonymous with mTBI: mTBI describes a type of injury whereas the post-concussion symptoms describe a set of problems presumably resulting from the injury.

It is particularly important to define clearly the patient's symptoms, as well as the course and resolution (or lack thereof) of those symptoms since the time of injury. Documenting frequency and severity of symptoms is important to set a baseline for monitoring subsequent treatment efficacy or establishment of co-occurring conditions. (See Table B-1)

Patients should be asked about the impact of their symptoms on their daily function. Individuals with a concussion/mTBI are typically independent in basic activities of daily living (ADLs) (e.g., grooming, bathing, dressing, toileting, and mobility). However, a small minority of patients may present with problems in areas of instrumental ADLs (IADLs). These abilities may affect independent functioning in tasks such as driving, home management, childcare, financial management, and performance at work.

Patients with symptoms should be asked open-ended questions to allow them to describe their difficulties. Presenting patients with symptom checklists is not recommended, however these lists may be useful in documenting symptoms and symptom intensity.

Patient Perception of Symptoms: Patients should be given the opportunity to relate their experiences and complaints at each visit in their own way. Although time-consuming and likely to include much seemingly irrelevant information, this has the advantage of providing considerable information concerning the patient's intelligence, emotional make-up, and attitudes about their complaints. This also provides patients with the satisfaction that they have been "heard-out" by the clinician, rather than merely being asked a few questions and exposed to a series of laboratory tests.

As the patient relates the history, important nonverbal clues are often provided. The clinician should observe the patient's attitude, reactions, and gestures while being questioned, as well as his or her choice of words or emphasis. The impact from the symptoms may range from annoying to totally disabling and patient perceptions regarding the cause and impact are important to understand in managing the disorder. Stressors such as occupational and family issues should also be explored.

Recommendations:

1) Self-reported symptomatology is an appropriate assessment of the patient's condition in concussion/mTBI when the history is consistent with having sustained an injury event and having a subsequent alteration in consciousness. [SR = C]
2) Assessment of the patient with concussion/mTBI should include detailed questioning about the frequency, intensity and nature of symptoms the patient experiences, and their impact on the patient's social and occupational functioning.
3) Assessment should include a review of all prescribed medications and over-the-counter supplements for possible causative or exacerbating influences. These should include caffeine, tobacco and other stimulants, such as energy drinks.
4) The patient who sustained a concussion/mTBI should be assessed for sleep patterns and sleep hygiene.
5) If the patient's symptoms significantly impact daily activities (such as child care, safe driving), a referral to rehabilitation specialists for a functional evaluation and treatment should be considered.

Discussion

Clarify the Symptoms: Questions that may prompt patients to provide important attributes of their symptoms are summarized in the following table.

Evidence Statements: *Is there a relationship between self-awareness and response to treatment of cognitive and psychological deficits in individuals with concussion/mTBI?*

Out of 40 studies identified in the initial search addressing self-reporting in mTBI, seven studies were found relevant to mild-TBI and of scientific quality.

Table B-1. Clarification of Symptoms

Symptom Attributes	Questions
Duration	o Has the symptom existed for days, weeks, or months? o Has the symptom occurred only intermittently? o Particularly with regard to pain and fatigue, can the patient define if these symptoms occurred only two or three days per month or constantly? o Is the symptom seasonal? o Are there times of the day when the symptom is worse?
Onset	o Can the patient recall exactly how the symptom began? o Were there triggering events, either physical or emotional? o Was the onset subtle and gradual, or dramatic and sudden? o Have the triggering events tended to be the same over time or are there changing patterns?
Location	o Is the symptom localized or diffuse? o Can the patient localize the symptom by pointing to it? o If the pain is diffuse, does it involve more than one body quadrant?
Co-morbidity	o Does the patient have any diagnosed co-existing illnesses? o What is the time relationship between the onset and severity of the co-existing illnesses and the symptoms of fatigue and/or pain? o What are the symptoms other than pain and/or fatigue? o Are there co-morbid diagnoses? o Are there changes in the patient's weight, mood, or diet?
Previous episodes	o If the symptoms are episodic, what is the pattern in regard to timing, intensity, triggering events, and response to any prior treatment?
Intensity and impact	o How severe are the symptoms (use the 1 to 10 Numerical Rating Scale) o Ask the patient to describe any new limitations they have experienced compared to their usual life-style, including limitations in physical endurance or strength (e.g., climbing stairs, shopping, and amount or quality of their sleep).
Previous treatment and medications	o Exploring this aspect of the history may be complicated and require obtaining prior medical records, or having an authorized telephone conversation with the prior treating clinician. o Ask the patient to bring in their medication bottles on a subsequent visit and document the exact names of the medications. o Find out which medications have/have not been helpful.
Past medical, surgical and psychological history	o This area includes chronic and major acute illnesses and injuries, allergies, surgical procedures, and hospitalizations. The psychological history may take several visits to clarify, depending upon the ease with which the patient can articulate their emotional status and past and present issues. Explore stressors such as occupational and family issues.
Patient perception of symptoms	o Often omitted from the history-taking are questions designed to gain some understanding of what the patient believes is happening. Ask the patient about their hunches and fears.

Unlike patients with more severe TBI, patients with concussion/mTBI are aware of their symptoms and can report these to providers. However, symptom-reporting is subjective by nature, and some patient reporting may not correspond with observed or objective findings.

- Use of self-reported symptomatology in post-concussion/mTBI is an appropriate assessment methodology, although comorbid mental health or socio-economic status conditions can undermine its reliability (Dirette et al., 2007; Gunstad & Suhr., 2001; Malec et al., 2007; Stulemeijer et al., 2007; Uomoto et al., 2004). (SR = C)
- Mild TBI is not associated with any reduced awareness of symptoms or problems (Dirette et al., 2007; Malec et al., 2007; Pagulayan et al., 2007; Stulemeijer et al., 2007; Uomoto et al., 2004)

- Some individuals with mTBI over-report symptoms. Over-reporting is associated with comorbid mental health conditions and lower levels of education (Gunstad & Suhr., 2001; Stuhlemeijer et al., 2007; Uomoto et al., 2004).
- Self-reported cognitive complaints are more strongly related to premorbid traits and physical and emotional state factors than to actual cognitive impairments (Gunstad & Suhr., 2001; Stulemeijer et al., 2007; Uomoto et al., 2004).

Annotation B-4 *Build Therapeutic Alliance*

Background: Interactions with patients/ families that involve real or suspected mTBI may be highly emotional, with reactions ranging from disbelief to anger to frustration to relief. Some patients will present with diagnosable symptoms, while others may believe they're suffering from mTBI when subsequent medical assessments may indicate otherwise. In both situations, medical staffs face the difficult challenge of effectively communicating the diagnosis, treatment, and prognosis for recovery to patients/ families, while minimizing and/or avoiding undue anxiety.

The information provided by medical personnel to individuals who have experienced a concussion/mTBI can either amplify and increase their symptoms and distress (iatrogenic factors), or can minimize and normalize their symptoms and reduce distress.

The lack of a definitive diagnosis or single effective treatment can make the management of patients with concussion/mTBI symptoms challenging and may also cause frustration for both the patient and the provider. To counter this, a high level of patient trust and faith in the clinician is required in order to maintain continuity of care and continue patient management through regular follow-up appointments. A therapeutic alliance between the patient and clinician should be established during the initial evaluation.

Risk communication approaches include:

1) **Caring and empathy**, including perceived sincerity, ability to listen, and to see issues from the perspective of others. Of the four factors, patient perceptions of caring and empathy are the most important.
2) **Competence and expertise**, including perceived intelligence, training, experience, education level, professional attainment, knowledge, and command of information. These are the easiest factors to establish because health care providers are automatically perceived by the public to be credible sources of information.
3) **Dedication and commitment**, including perceived altruism, diligence, self-identification, involvement, and hard work. Perceptions of dedication and commitment are influenced by patient perceptions of the health care provider's hard work in the pursuit of health goals.
4) **Honesty and openness**, including perceived truthfulness, candidness, fairness, objectivity, and sincerity. Perceptions of this factor result from both nonverbal cues (i.e., posture, eye contact, facial expressions, interruptions, indirect language) and language that convey sincerity and concern. Sensitivity to nonverbal cues is especially invaluable in ultimately understanding and communicating effectively with the patient and their family.

Useful strategies to strengthen the partnership with the patient:

- Acknowledge and indicate commitment to understand the patient's concerns and symptoms
- Encourage an open and honest transfer of information that will provide a more comprehensive picture of the patient's concerns and medical history
- Present information regarding a positive outcome and symptom remission to create an expectation of recovery
- Indicate commitment to allocate sufficient time and resources to resolving the patient's concerns
- Avoid open skepticism or disapproving comments in discussing the patient's concerns
- At each patient visit, the clinician should consider the following:
  - Ask if there are unaddressed or unresolved concerns
  - Summarize and explain all test results
  - Schedule follow-up visits in a timely manner
  - Explain that outstanding or interim consultations will be reviewed during the follow-up visits
  - Offer to include the concerned family member or significant other in the follow-up visit.

Research has shown that the quality of health care provider-patient communications can critically influence the quality of life for patients and families, as well as patient health outcomes. Risk communication techniques (See Appendix C: Health Risk Communication) have been demonstrated as effective for providers in communicating with patients with diagnosed or suspected concussion/mTBI and their families. Regardless of the diagnosis, medical staff must communicate "bad news" in a manner that clearly communicates the necessary medical information, while balancing the physical, emotional, and social needs of the patient/ family. The ability to do this successfully requires excellent and well-practiced risk communication skills. It is important to note that even when risk communication is effective, not all conflicts can be resolved.

Annotation B-5 *Determine Treatment Plan*

4 .Treatment

4.1. Treatment Plan

Background: After the screening, assessment, and diagnosis of concussion/mTBI are completed decisions are made about treatment. Treatment for patients with concussion/mTBI focuses on symptom management and education of patient and family. Education should emphasize recovery, gradual resumption of work and social responsibilities, and teaching compensatory strategies and environmental modifications. Most patients with symptoms following a single concussion/mTBI of recent onset can be successfully managed in the primary care setting without the need for specialty intervention.

Patients should be encouraged to implement changes in life-style including exercise, diet, sleep hygiene, stress reduction, relaxation training, scheduling leisure activities and pacing to improve treatment outcomes.

Recommendations:

1) Develop and document a summary of the patient's problems.
2) Develop a potential treatment plan that includes severity and urgency for treatment interventions.
3) Discuss with the patient the general concept of concussion sequelae, treatment options and associated risk/benefits and prognosis of illness to determine the patient's preferences.
4) Emphasizing good prognosis and empowering the patient for self-management,
5) Implement the treatment plan and follow up.
6) Referral to specialty care is not required in the majority of patients with concussion/mTBI, if their symptoms resolve in the early post acute recovery period as expected.
7) Treatment should be coordinated and may include consultation with rehabilitation therapists, pharmacy, collaborative mental health, and social support.

Discussion: The need for a consistent and cohesive approach by an interdisciplinary team is paramount when treating persons with the cognitive and behavioral impairments that can occur with concussion/mTBI. The interdisciplinary team is made up of practitioners from multiple disciplines that function collaboratively to achieve common objectives. The team determines specific interventions based on analysis of the assessment information with feedback from all team members including the patient and caregiver(s). Interventions are formalized into an individualized plan of care with specific long-term goals, short-term objectives. Both the persons with concussion/mTBI and their support system should be active participants in the process of developing and reviewing the treatment plan.

Role of the Provider in the Initial Care Setting: The provider in the initial setting of care should develop a problem list that summarizes the patient's problems. The provider should determine the severity of each identified problem and the impact it will have on the patient's functional ability and quality of life, so that a baseline can be established against which improvements can be assessed.

The provider should also identify problems for which treatment is most urgently recommended.

The most urgent treatments may be defined as those treatments expected to result in the greatest improvement when addressing the most severe problems.

Treatment Interventions: Cost-effective interventions (e.g., giving the patient an information booklet about symptoms and coping strategies, a telephone follow-up, or "as-needed services") were effective in alleviating chronic symptom development (Mittenberg et al., 1996; Paniak et al., 2000; Ponsford, 2005).

Still, other healthcare professionals suggest that cognitive rehabilitation and emotional support are likely to improve the outcomes for persons with mTBI (Paniak et al.; Tiersky et al., 2005).

Components of Patient Education

- Provision of information about concussion/mTBI
- Strategies for prevention of further injury
- Education/normalization
- Awareness of limitation
- Self-monitoring ofsymptoms
- Contact information.

Cicerone and associates' review (2005) found that neuropsychological rehabilitation therapies involving combination therapies for persons with cognitive, emotional, interpersonal, and motivational deficits are usually focused on those with moderate to severe brain trauma.

Although there is evidence that rehabilitation is beneficial for improving community integration and return to work for persons with moderate-to-severe injuries, this evidence is *not* available for those with milder injuries.

Research concerning optimal treatment for those with mTBI suggests that less expensive approaches may be effective and that the more comprehensive, multidisciplinary treatment should be targeted toward those with pre-injury psychiatric problems (Ghaffar et al., 2006).

Annotation B-6 *Educate Patient/Family on Symptoms and Expected Recovery of Concussion/mTBI*

4.2. Early Education

Background: Education provided to patients and their support system about the nature and common manifestations of concussion/mTBI is a critical aspect of intervention. Communication of health information from providers helps manage patient expectations and can prevent the development of concussion/mTBI symptoms and/or reduce their duration, number, and severity. It is generally recommended that the initial educational intervention occur at the time of establishing the concussion/mTBI diagnosis. Follow-up education should take place at intervals and in a format that is appropriate to the treatment and services provided. Additionally, the patient's learning needs, reading skills, vision or hearing difficulties, cultural and religious beliefs, and emotional or cognitive limitations should be taken into consideration when delivering educational information.

Recommendations:

1. Patients who sustain a concussion/mTBI should be provided with information and education about concussion/mTBI symptoms and recovery patterns as soon as possible after the injury. Education should be provided in printed material combined with verbal review and consist of:

a) Symptoms and expected outcome [SR = A]
b) Normalizing symptoms (education that current symptoms are expected and common after injury event) [SR = A]
c) Reassurance about expected positive recovery [SR = A]

d) Techniques to manage stress (e.g., sleep education, relaxation techniques; minimize consumption of alcohol, caffeine and other stimulants). [SR = B]

2. Information and education should also be offered to the patient's family, friends, employers, and/or significant others.

3. Symptomatic management should include tailored education about the specific signs and symptoms that the patient presents and the recommended treatment.

4. Patients should be provided with written contact information and be advised to contact their healthcare provider for follow-up if their condition deteriorates or if symptoms persist for more than 4-6 weeks. [SR = B]

Rationale: Fears and misconceptions of the injury and its sequelae can amplify or sustain symptoms and result in poor outcomes. The observation that patients respond positively across most symptom domains to appropriate information and reassurance given shortly after injury, suggests that an early educational intervention can speed the recovery and decreases the severity of post concussion symptoms.

Evidence Statements: *Does early intervention education decrease the incidence and severity of chronic concussion/mTBI symptoms and lead to better outcomes?*

The Working Group reviewed abstracts of nineteen articles published since 2002. One systematic review of randomized trials and one individual study assessing the efficacy of early education that were not included in the WHO task force project were identified. In the final analysis, based on two systematic reviews (Borg 2004, Comper 2005), there is strong evidence to recommend early educational intervention for patients with concussion/mTBI.

- Borg (2004) in assessing the WHO findings referenced five studies (Paniak et al, 1998, Paniak et al 2000, Wade et al 1997, Wade et al., 1998; Mittenberg 1996) that supported the idea that a single session intervention was as effective as more elaborate assessments and interventions. The WHO Task Force did not find strong evidence that any non-surgical treatment has a clinically important effect on symptoms or disability after mTBI but that a few studies on early intervention provided some evidence that early, limited, educational intervention reduces long-term complaints. The task force recommended that early, structured, educational information in connection with acute care or within one week after should be provided to patients with uncomplicated mTBI; information about the injury, about common complaints and how to cope with them, reassurance about a good outcome, and information on how to get access to further support when needed should be included and these patients should be encouraged to become active as soon as possible after their injury.
- Comper (2005) in a systematic review included seven trials (Paniak 1998, 2000, Hinkle 1986, Mittenberg, 2001, Ponsford, 2002, Wade 1997, 1998) assessing the efficacy or information provision intervention. The review found that there is sufficient evidence to support patient-centered interaction and the provision of symptom-related information through treating practitioners as effective in assisting individuals in their recovery from concussion/mTBI. The three studies that compared minimal and intensive education interventions found consistent evidence that brief

educational and reassurance-oriented intervention is as effective as a potentially more intensive and expensive educational model. The four studies that compared an educational intervention to usual hospital services found that patients who received an enhanced level of care including print educational materials experienced fewer or less severe PCS symptoms and less disruption of social and functioning ability than patients who received usual hospital care. In most studies, simple education and support appeared to benefit individuals with concussion/mTBI with respect to somatic and psychological complaints.

- Provision of educational information regarding the common symptoms of mTBI and the expected and typical positive prognosis, reduces symptom intensity and duration (Mittenberg et al., 1996; Ponsford et al., 2002).
- Printed educational material alone may not be helpful (Gronwall, 1986), but printed material combined with verbal review has been shown in multiple studies to be helpful.
- Teaching stress and symptom self-management techniques may be useful in reducing symptom intensity and duration, particularly in combination with other educational and normalization interventions (Mittenberg et al., 1996).

Annotation B-7 *Provide Early Interventions*

4.3. Provide Early Intervention

Background: Concussion/mTBI can significantly impact some patients' physical, mental and social well-being. Treatment should address these three main areas. Initial interventions expected to improve physical well-being include education, improved sleep habits, a graduated exercise regimen (monitored through physical therapy, exercise trainers, and social supports), and medication (monitored by a clinician). Mental wellbeing may be improved through stress relief and relaxation, medication, and creating a supportive social network. Social well-being may be improved through resolving legal, financial, occupational, or recreational problems.

Recommendations:

1. Provide early intervention maximizing the use of non-pharmacological therapies:

a) Review sleep patterns and hygiene and provide sleep education including education about excess use of caffeine/tobacco/alcohol and other stimulants

b) Recommend graded aerobic exercise with close monitoring.

4.4. Return to Activity (Duty/Work/School/Leisure)

Background: A successful treatment outcome for a patient who has sustained a concussion is the return to duty/work/school or other usual daily activities. Part of the early intervention for concussion/mTBI involves protecting the patient from a secondary insult or further injury by limiting or eliminating their duty status or job requirements until proper recovery is obtained. Although rare, the possibility of second impact syndrome must be prevented by altering a concussed patient's vocational duties when they are high risk for re-injury. Exertional testing prior to the return to work or military duty may help to ensure adequate resolution of symptoms in a high stress state or combat environment.

Return to activity assessment is based on an inventory of symptoms and their severity and the patient's job-specific tasks. With the exception of those activities and duties that are characterized as high-risk for repeat concussions, all individuals with concussion/mTBI should be encouraged to expediently return to activity at their maximum capacity.

Activity restrictions are an important part of the treatment regimen for patients with concussion/mTBI.

Activity restriction *does not imply complete bed rest but rather a restful pattern of activity throughout the day with minimal physical and mental exertion.*

Recommendations:

1) Immediately following any concussion/mTBI, individuals who present with post-injury symptoms should have a period of rest to avoid sustaining another concussion and to facilitate a prompt recovery.
2) Individuals with concussion/mTBI should be encouraged to expediently return to normal activity (work, school, duty, leisure) at their maximal capacity.
3) In individuals who report symptoms of fatigue, consideration should be given to a graded return to work/activity.
4) In instances where there is high risk for injury and/or the possibility of duty-specific tasks that cannot be safely or competently completed, an assessment of the symptoms and necessary needs for accommodations should be conducted through a focused interview and examination of the patient.
5) If a person's normal activity involves significant physical activity, exertional testing can be conducted that includes stressing the body.
6) If exertional testing results in a return of symptoms, a monitored progressive return to normal activity as tolerated should be recommended.
7) Individually based work duty restriction should apply if:
   - There is a duty specific task that cannot be safely or competently completed based on symptoms
   - The work/duty environment cannot be adapted to the patient's symptom-based limitation
   - The deficits cannot be accommodated
   - Symptoms reoccur.

Rationale: There is limited utility in using the sports related return to play guidelines or research to make return to work determinations.

The purpose of most sport studies is to predict subsequent concussion rather than recovery of symptoms or health outcomes. In the sports arena, there is an opportunity to observe the concussion and continuously monitor the players including access for pre- and post-injury function assessment.

The uniqueness of these characteristics does not allow generalizing the conclusions of sport research to the clinical setting.

In the lack of evidence, the Working Group concluded that with the exception of those individuals returning to activity/duty with a high repeat concussion risk, all individuals with concussion/mTBI should be encouraged to expediently return to work at their maximal capacity.

Return to activity assessment is based on an inventory of symptoms and job-specific tasks. There is no available research to support the validity or utility of physical, cognitive or behavioral stress testing as a predictor of ability to return to activity/duty following concussion/mTBI. Physical exertional testing for evaluating readiness has not been shown to cause harm in patients with concussion/mTBI.

Evidence Statements: *What are the key factors in successful return to work in individuals with concussion/mTBI?*

There has been no research evidence that early return to work after concussion/mTBI with or without symptoms is detrimental. Most of the literature regarding criteria for return to activities after concussion has been focused on sports medicine and return to play. Sports organizations have developed return to play guidelines, however these were consensus based. Research evidence supports that a sports-specific stepwise return to play program after resolution of symptoms is recommended in sports concussion (Kissick & Johnston, 2005].

- Current guidelines for grading sports-related concussions base their return-to-play recommendations largely on two parameters: the severity of the injury and the patient's history of concussion.
- The two most widely used guidelines are those of the American Association of Neurological Surgeons (AANS) and those of Cantu. Both guidelines use a grading system to assess the injury severity that takes into account the nature and duration of key injury characteristics. Concussion is graded as I (mild), II (moderate), and III (severe). The AAN guidelines emphasize the qualitative importance of loss of consciousness (LOC), whereas Cantu guidelines (1986; 1998) distinguish between brief and extended LOC, and draw attention to the duration of posttraumatic amnesia.
- According to the Cantu Guidelines, athletes with Grade I concussions may return to play if no symptoms are present for one week.
- Grade II concussion involves loss of consciousness for less than five minutes or exhibit posttraumatic amnesia between 30 minutes and 24 hours in duration. Players who sustain this grade of concussion may also return to play after one week of being asymptomatic.
- Grade III concussions involve posttraumatic amnesia for more than 24 hours or unconsciousness for more than five minutes. Players who sustain this grade of concussion should be sidelined for at least one month, after which they can return to play if they are asymptomatic for one week.
- The guideline recommendation for complete cessation of symptoms before return-to-play is not based on evidence of harm in those who continue to play with persistent symptoms, nor is it based on evidence of lack of harm in athletes who play after their symptoms have completely resolved (Peloso et al., 2004).
- Following repeated concussions, a player should be sidelined for longer periods of time and possibly not allowed to play for the remainder of the season.

Annotation B-8 Initiate Symptom-Based Treatment Modalities

5. Symptom Management

Concussion/mTBI is associated with a variety of symptoms that will manifest immediately following the event, and may resolve quickly, within minutes to hours after the injury event, or they may persist longer. Signs and symptoms may occur alone or in varying combinations and may result in functional impairment.

The most typical signs and symptoms following concussion include:

a) Physical: headache, nausea, vomiting, dizziness, fatigue, blurred vision, sleep disturbance, sensitivity to light/noise, balance problems, transient neurological abnormalities
b) Cognitive: attention, concentration, memory, speed of processing, judgment, executive control
c) Behavioral/emotional: depression, anxiety, agitation, irritability, impulsivity, aggression.

There is a complex relationship among concussion/mTBI symptoms (sleep, headache, cognition, and mood) and it is clinically reasonable to expect that alleviating/improving one symptom may lead to improvement in other symptom clusters. The presence of comorbid psychiatric problems such as a major depressive episode, anxiety disorders (including post-traumatic stress disorder [PTSD]), or substance use disorder (SUD) – whether or not these are regarded as etiologically related to the concussion/mTBI – should be treated aggressively using appropriate psychotherapeutic and pharmacologic interventions.

The expected outcome of intervention should be to improve the identified problem areas, rather than discover a disease etiology or "cure." The persistence of some concussion related symptoms despite the effective treatment for others does not necessarily suggest treatment failure, but may instead indicate the need for additional therapies targeting specific residual symptoms.

The following recommended interventions focus on initial management of the physical, cognitive and behavioral symptoms.

Patients with symptoms that persist despite these initial treatment interventions should be managed using **Algorithm C: Follow-up Persistent symptoms**

5.1. Physical Symptoms

Background: For purposes of this guideline, physical complaints include headache, pain, sleep disturbances, dizziness, coordination issues, nausea, numbness, smell/taste, vision difficulties (photophobia, phonophobia), hearing difficulties, fatigue, and appetite disturbances.

In the majority of cases, these symptoms are markedly improved or have disappeared within 3 months after the injury.

Recommendations:

1. Initial treatment of physical complaints of a patient with concussion/mTBI should be based upon a thorough evaluation, individual factors and symptom presentation.

2. The evaluation should include:

a) Establishing a thorough medical history, completing a physical examination, and review of the medical record (for specific components for each symptoms see Table B-2 Physical Symptoms-Assessment)
b) Minimizing low yield diagnostic testing
c) Identifying treatable causes (conditions) for patient's symptoms
d) Referring for further evaluation as appropriate.

3. The treatment should include:

a) Non-pharmacological interventions such as sleep hygiene education, physical therapy, relaxation and modification of the environment (for specific components for each symptoms see Table B-3 Physical Symptoms-Treatment)
b) Use of medications to relieve pain, enable sleep, relaxation and stress reduction.

4. A consultation or referral to specialists for further assessment should occur when:
a) Symptoms cannot be linked to a concussion event (suspicion of another diagnosis)
b) An atypical symptom pattern or course is present
c) Findings indicate an acute neurologic condition that requires urgent neurologic/neurosurgical intervention (see Section 3.1.2 – Physical Examination)
d) There are other major co-morbid conditions requiring special evaluation.

Evidence Statements:

- The WHO task force did not find strong evidence that any non-surgical treatment has a clinically important effect on symptoms or disability after mTBI (Borg, 2004).
  The review of the literature since the report of the WHO task force did not reveal any research evidence to support the role of specific interventions to improve any of the somatic (physical) complaints after concussion/mTBI.
- Self reported symptoms are common after concussion/mTBI; however there is little consistency in findings about how long such symptoms persist.
  The stronger studies of mTBI that use appropriate control groups and consider the effects of other non-mTBI factors generally show resolution of symptoms within weeks or a few months (Holm, 2005).
- Several uncontrolled and/or observational studies found the following physical symptoms are reported by persons after a concussion/mTBI:
  - Headache (See Appendix D)
  - Dizziness (Ernst et al., 2005; Hoffer et al., 2004; Staab et al., 2007) - Acute and persistent. [SR = I] (See Appendix D)
  - Upper and lower extremity coordination (Catena et al., 2007; Heitger et al., 2006; Parker et al., 2006) - Acute and persistent. [SR=I] (See Appendix D)
  - Sleep (Chaput et al., 2007; Mahmood et al., 2004; Oullette et al., 2006), acute and persistent [SR = C] (See Appendix D)
  - Fatigue (Borgaro et al., 2005; Stulemeijer et al., 2006), persistent [SR = I] (See Appendix D)
  - Hearing: Persistent [SR=C]
    - Hyperaccusis, tinnitus, auditory acuity deficits, auditory processing disorders (Nolle, 2004)

- Vision:
    - Visual tracking (saccades) (Dehaan et al., 2007; Heitger et al., 2004; Suh et al., 2006; Suh et al., 2006), acute and persistent [SR = C]
    - Visual attention (Dehaan et al., 2007; Halterman et al., 2006; Tinius et al., 2003), acute and persistent [SR = C]
- There is inconsistent evidence to support the association of concussion/mTBI with the following symptoms during the initial presentation for post-concussive symptoms, although some patients may still report them:
    - Numbness
    - Appetite disturbance
    - Nausea
    - Smell
- Research evidence supports that auditory symptoms may improve more rapidly than physiologic measures of auditory function (Nolle et al., 2004).
- Multiple non-TBI related factors can also be associated with above symptoms:
    - Sleep (Chaput, et al., 2007; Oullette et al., 2006)
    - Vision (Heitger et al., 2004)
    - Fatigue (Stulemeijer et al., 2006; Ziino et al., 2005)

5.2. Cognitive Symptoms

Background: Although initial cognitive complaints and problems are common in the first hours and days after a concussion/mTBI, the vast majority of individuals recover within one to four weeks.

Early psychoeducational, supportive, and stress management interventions have been shown to increase rate and extent of recovery from somatic, cognitive and behavioral symptoms. As rapid recovery is expected, patients should always be provided with positive expectations.

See Table B-4: Behavioral and Cognitive Symptoms – ASSESSMENT and B-5: Behavioral and Cognitive Symptoms – TREATMENT

Recommendations:

1) All individuals who sustain a concussion/mTBI should be provided with information and education about concussion/mTBI symptoms and recovery patterns as soon as possible after the injury [SR = A] (See Early Education, Section 4.2)
2) A patient sustaining a concussion/mTBI should be evaluated for cognitive difficulties using a focused clinical interview. [SR = C]
3) Comprehensive neuropsychological/cognitive testing is not recommended during the first 30 days post injury. [SR = D]
4) If a pre-injury neurocognitive baseline was established in an individual case, then a post injury comparison may be completed by a psychologist but should be determined using reliable tools and test-retest stability should be ensured. [SR = B]

Evidence Statements: *Are there cognitive rehabilitation techniques that have been shown to result in better outcomes in individuals with concussion/mTBI?*

The working group reviewed 23 studies related to cognitive factors associated with concussion/mTBI that were published after 2002.

However, none were found acceptable for the purpose of this guideline.

Most addressed patients with moderate or severe TBI, or did not provide evidence related to the question. Several older studies that are included were referenced in the systematic review published by Comper et al., (2005) and three meta-analyses (Belanger et al., 2005; Belanger & Vanderploeg, 2005; Schretlen & Shapiro, 2003).

Table B-2. Physical Symptoms – ASSESSMENT

Common Symptoms Following Concussion/mTBI *	Meds Review	Assess for HTN	Physical Examination					Sleep Review	Depression Screen	Differential Diagnoses Include:
			GI	Neuro	Musc	Vision	Otological			
Headaches	√	√		√	√	√	√	√		*Pre-existing headache disorder (migraine, tension)* *Cervical spine or musculature abnormality or pain CSF leak or pressure abnormality* *Sinus infection* *Visual acuity issues (needs glasses)*
Feeling dizzy - Loss of balance - Poor coordination - Clumsy	√			√	√	√	√			*Inner ear infection* *Labyrinthitis* *CSF leak or pressure abnormality Meniere's disease Orthostatic hypotension Central medication effect*
Nausea	√		√		√	√	√			*GI ulcer GERD* *Medication effect*
Change in appetite	√		√							*Nasal polyps Sinus infection* *Traumatic injury to olfactory or lingual nerves*
Sleep disturbance - Difficulty falling or staying a sleep (insomnia)	√							√	√	*Behavioral health issues Sleep disorders Pain*
Vision problems - Blurring - Trouble seeing - Sensitivity to light	√				√	√	√	√		*Retinal detachment Traumatic injury to lens Corneal abrasion Optic nerve damage*
Hearing difficulty - Sensitivity to noise	√						√			*Inner ear infection Ear drum inflammation Ear drum injury Traumatic auditory nerve injury*

Other less common symptoms following concussion/mTBI include:

- **Numbness or tingling on parts of the body** – Review of medications, neurological exam and EMG to rule out *stroke, multiple sclerosis, spinal cord injury, peripheral neuropathy, or thoracic outlet syndrome* - **Change in taste and/or smell** – neurological exam to rule out nasal polyps, sinus infection, or traumatic injury to olfactory or lingual nerves.

Table B-3. Physical Symptoms – Treatment

Common Symptoms Following Concussion/mTBI	Pharmacologic Treatment	Non-Pharmacologic Treatment
Headaches	- Non narcotic pain meds - NSAIDs - Triptans (migraine type)	- Sleep hygiene education - Physical therapy - Relaxation
Feeling dizzy	- Antibiotics, decongestants for infections and fluid	- -
Loss of balance Poor coordination	-	- Physical therapy
Nausea	- Antiemetics	- Sleep hygiene education
Change in appetite	-	-
Sleep disturbances - Difficulty falling or staying asleep (insomnia)	- Sleep Medications	- Sleep hygiene education
Vision problems - Blurring - Trouble seeing - Sensitivity to light	-	- Sleep hygiene education - Light desensitization - Sunglasses
Hearing difficulty - Sensitivity to noise	-	- Environmental Modifications

- Under standardized and controlled conditions and using reliable instruments, initial cognitive decline and subsequent recovery have been demonstrated by comparing base-line assessment to post-injury assessment of cognitive performance in athletes (Macciocchi et al., 1996; McCrea et al., 2003; McCrea et al., 2002).
- There is good evidence from three meta-analyses that cognitive performance declines in the immediate period after a concussion/m/TBI injury (initial 7-30 days). Studies have demonstrated initial cognitive impairments using standardized and valid measuring instrument (Belanger et al., 2005; Belanger & Vanderploeg, 2005; Schretlen & Shapiro, 2003).
- Cognitive impairment in the initial 7 – 30 days has been demonstrated in the following domains; memory, complex attention or working memory, and speed of mental and motor performance (including verbal and non-verbal generative tasks) (Belanger et al., 2005; Belanger & Vanderploeg, 2005).
- Group data shows resolution of cognitive problems in most patients in 7 –30 days after injury (Belanger et al., 2005; Belanger & Vanderploeg, 2005; Schretlen & Shapiro, 2003).
- Some studies show that a subgroup of individuals continue to have both subjective symptoms (Alves et al., 1993; Deb et al., 1999; Dikmen et al., 1986; Hartlage et al., 2001; Luis et al., 2003; Powell et al., 1996) and lower cognitive test performance even after 90 days (Belanger et al., 2005; Binder et al., 1997; Vanderploeg et al., 2005).
- In the acute phase of recovery brief psychoeducational, supportive, stress management, and/or cognitive-behavioral interventions have consistently been

shown to result in improvement in subjective complaints including cognitive issues (Anson & Ponsford, 2006; Bédard et al. 2002, Mittenberg et al., 1996, Hinkle et al., 1986; Comper et al., 2005)

- The relationship between subjective complaints and test performance is complex. There is more correlation in the acute phase than post-acute phase.
- There is limited evidence for the diagnostic validity of cognitive testing and other diagnostic tools for mild traumatic brain injury (Cassidy et al., 2004).

5.3. Behavioral Symptoms

Background: Depending upon diagnostic criteria (ICD-9 versus DSM-IV) the following behavioral or personality changes may be considered part of the post-concussion syndrome: irritability, depression, anxiety, emotional lability, fatigue, insomnia, reduced alcohol tolerance, personality changes such as increases in socially inappropriate behaviors, and apathy or lack of spontaneity.

Anxiety and depression and other mental health problems also have been associated with concussion/mTBI.

The presence of comorbid psychiatric problems such as a major depressive episode, anxiety disorders (including post-traumatic stress disorder), or substance abuse – whether or not these are regarded as etiologically related to the mild TBI – should be treated aggressively using appropriate psychotherapeutic and pharmacologic interventions.

See Table B-4: Behavioral and Cognitive Symptoms – ASSESSMENT and B-5: Behavioral and Cognitive Symptoms – TREATMENT

Recommendations:

1) Patients with concussion/mTBI should be screened for psychiatric symptoms and co-morbid psychiatric disorders (Depression, Post Traumatic Stress, and Substance Use).
2) Treatment of psychiatric/behavioral symptoms following concussion/mTBI should be based upon individual factors and nature and severity of symptom presentation, and include both psychotherapeutic [SR = A] and pharmacological [SR = I] treatment modalities.
3) Individuals who sustain a concussion/mTBI and present with anxiety symptoms and/or irritability should be provided reassurance regarding recovery and offered a several week trial of pharmacologic agents (See Appendix E) .[SR = I]

Evidence Statements:

- There is considerable evidence that several psychiatric conditions are associated with mTBI – specifically affective disorders (Fann, 2004; McCauley et al., 2001; Suhr, 2002), combat-stress spectrum disorders (Hoge et al., 2008; McCauley, et al., 2001; Moore, 2006) and some association with Substance Use Disorder(Carroll, 2004; Horner, 2005; Parry-Jones, 2004).
- There is some support for the effectiveness of treating post-traumatic stress symptomatology following mTBI using cognitive-behavioral therapy (Bryant et al., 2003; Soo & Tate, 2007), as well as a combination of cognitive-behavioral therapy and neuropsychological rehabilitation (Soo & Tate, 2007; Tiersky et al., 2005).

- Co-morbid depression or other mental disorders are associated with higher rates of persistent post-concussive symptoms and poorer outcomes following concussion/mTBI (Iverson, 2006; Mooney et al., 2001; Rapoport, 2006).

Table B-4. Behavioral and Cognitive Symptoms – ASSESSMENT

Common Symptoms Following Concussion/mTBI	Review Medications	Lab Tests: Electrolytes CBC TFT	Review Sleep Habits	Screen for: - Depression - PTSD - SUD	Differential Diagnosis or Comorbid Conditions Include:
Fatigue - Loss of energy - Getting tired easily	√	√	√	√	*- Anxiety disorders* *- Chronic Fatigue Syndrome* *- Chronic pain* *- Depression or other mood disorders* *- Insomnia* *- Metabolic disorders* *- Sleep Apnea* *- Stress disorders* *- Substance use*
Cognitive difficulties – Concentration - Memory - Decision-making	√	√	√	√	
Feeling anxious	√	√	√	√	
Emotional difficulties - Feeling depressed - Irritability - Poor frustration tolerance	√	√	√	√	

Key: CBC-complete blood count; TFT-thyroid function test; PTSD-post-traumatic stress disorder; SUD-substance use disorder.

Table B-5. Behavioral and Cognitive Symptoms – TREATMENT

Common Symptoms Following Concussion/mTBI	Job Review	Pharmacologic Treatment	Non-Pharmacologic Treatment	Referral after failed response to initial intervention
Fatigue - Loss of energy - Getting tired easily	√	*	Reassurance Encourage regular scheduled aerobic exercise Activity restriction adjustment Sleep hygiene Education Sleep study	- Mental Health
Cognitive difficulties - Concentration - Memory - Decision-making	√	SSRI *		Consider referral to: - Cognitive rehabilitation - Mental Health - TBI specialist
Feeling anxious	√	Anxiolytic (short term) SSRI		- Mental Health - Social support
Emotional difficulties - Feeling depressed - Irritability - Poor frustration tolerance	√	Anti epileptics SSRI		

* Consider in the specialty care setting after ruling out a sleep disorder.

5.4. Pharmacotherapy

Background: At present, there is no clinically validated specific brain targeted pharmacotherapy that will ameliorate the neurocognitive effects attributed to TBI (e.g., enhancing memory and attention, recovering from the brain injury). No medication has received approval from the United States Food and Drug Administration (FDA) for the treatment of any neurological or psychiatric consequence of mTBI.

There are a number of effective adjunctive treatments for symptoms, that when used appropriately and cautiously can improve neurological and functional outcome. While there is little empiric evidence, some experts prescribe medications for attention, irritability, sleep, and mood disorders.

Table B-6. Considerations in Using Medication for Treatment of Symptoms

- Avoid medications that lower the seizure threshold (e.g., bupropion or traditional antipsychotic medications) or those that can cause confusion (e.g., lithium, benzodiazepines, anticholinergic agents).
- Before prescribing medications, rule out social factors (abuse, neglect, caregiver conflict, environmental issues).
- Unless side effects prevail, give full therapeutic trials at maximal tolerated doses before discontinuing a medication trial. Under-treatment is common. Start low and go slow with titration.
- Brain injured patients are more sensitive to side effects: watch closely for toxicity and drug-drug interactions.
- Limit quantities of medications with high risk for suicide as the suicide rate is higher in this population.
- Educate patients and family/care givers to avoid the use of alcohol with the medications.
- Minimize caffeine and avoid herbal, diet supplements such as "energy" products as some contain agents that cross-react with the psychiatric medications and lead to a hypertensive crisis.
- Avoid medications that contribute to cognitive slowing, fatigue or daytime drowsiness.

For suggested classes of medication treatment for specific symptoms, see Tables B-3 and B-5. For selected agents, dosages, and pharmacological data, see Appendix E.

Recommendations:

1) Medication for ameliorating the neurocognitive effects attributed to concussion/mTBI is not recommended.
2) Treatment of concussion/mTBI should be symptom-specific.
3) Medications may be considered for headaches, musculoskeletal pain, depression/anxiety, sleep disturbances, chronic fatigue or poor emotional control or lability.
4) Appropriate and aggressive pain management strategies should be employed.
5) When prescribing any medication for patients who have sustained a concussion/ mTBI, the following should be considered:
    a) Review and minimize all medication and over-the-counter supplements that may exacerbate or maintain symptoms
    b) Use caution when initiating new pharmacologic interventions to avoid the sedating properties that may have an impact upon a person's attention, cognition, and motor performance.

c) Recognize the risk of overdose with therapy of many medication classes (e.g., tricyclics). Initial quantities dispensed should reflect this concern.
d) Initiate therapy with the lowest effective dose, allow adequate time for any drug trials, and titrate dosage slowly based on tolerability and clinical response.
e) Document and inform all those who are treating the person of current medications and any medication changes.

Evidence Statement:

- The use of drugs in the treatment of various concussion/mTBI symptoms has not been studied in prospective studies. Thus, there is insufficient evidence to form specific recommendations.
- Medication(s) targeting any presumed underlying processes are not supported by the literature.
- In the absence of published studies with which to guide treatment, the selection of pharmacologic agents is based on expert opinion following the approach and experience used to select such agents for patients with cognitive, behavioral, or physical symptoms arising from other neurological or behavioral conditions.

5.5. Physical Rehabilitation

Background: Therapeutic exercise has been shown to positively impact the vast majority of disabilities. These exercises can be general and directed at an overall improvement in cardiopulmonary health, physical strength and power, and overall well-being; or focused at specific musculoskeletal, sensory or neuromuscular impairments that limit performance of daily activities. Following concussion/mTBI, those individuals that have persistent symptoms will often lapse in their overall conditioning. This will in turn result in a decrease in short- and long-term global health (physical and behavioral) and put them at an elevated risk for disability, pain, and handicap (i.e., difficulty with return to work, maintaining peer networks.)

Recommendations:

1) There is no contraindication for return to aerobic, fitness and therapeutic activities after concussion/mTBI. Non-contact, aerobic and recreational activities should be encouraged within the limits of the patient's symptoms to improve physical, cognitive and behavioral complaints and symptoms after concussion/mTBI. [SR = B]
2) Specific vestibular, visual, and proprioceptive therapeutic exercise is recommended for dizziness, disequilibrium, and spatial disorientation impairments after concussion/mTBI. (See Appendix D)
3) Specific therapeutic exercise is recommended for acute focal musculoskeletal impairments after concussion/mTBI.

5.5.1. General Exercise

Symptoms of concussion/mTBI amenable to general fitness programs are multiple somatic complaints without specific identified mechanisms of injury and an absence of physical findings.

The type of exercise (strength training, core stability, aerobic activities, ROM) is no different than those recommended for individuals without concussion/mTBI.

However, one should consider a gradual increase in duration and intensity due to the activity intolerance and fatigue that is commonly associated with concussion/mTBI. Implementation of a scheduled daily routine and incorporation of peer networks may improve compliance.

5.5.2. Focused Exercise

Focal impairments (e.g., upper cervical root entrapment, impaired gaze stability, oculomotor dysfunction) benefit from tailored exercise programs that promote adaptation of or compensation for the affected systems (vestibular, visual, and proprioceptive) or specific musculoskeletal/neuromuscular impairments (decreased ROM, weakness, timing).

The exercises that are commonly prescribed for these systems/impairments will be warranted. It is the delivery of instruction, guidance and follow-up needs that will be greater for those with mTBI.

As well, the duration and intensity level may need to be considered when looking at the overall presentation of the individual.

5.6. Alternative Modalities

Background: The vast majority of individuals with concussion/mTBI will have no difficulties or complaints following injury.

While early interventions have been shown to prevent and treat persistent somatic, cognitive and behavioral deficits, certain individuals will have persistent difficulties. Additionally, a significant percentage of individuals with concussion/mTBI will not receive early diagnosis or will not seek treatment, and therefore their symptoms will be addressed only after a temporal delay.

In many of these individuals with chronic persistent symptoms after mTBI, traditional medical interventions are less than successful.

Complementary alternative medicine (CAM) may be sought by the patient or patient's family. CAM interventions may assist in the treatment of certain symptoms associated with concussion/mTBI.

An evidence-based approach to the implementation of complementary medicine strategies will be useful to prevent over- or underutilization of CAM.

- Acupuncture
- Bio-feedback

Novel therapy (hyperbaric oxygen, nutritional supplements) modalities in the management of concussion/mTBI are being explored in the field as potential treatment approaches.

It is the recommendation of the Working Group that interventions which lack sufficient empirical support should occur only under the auspices of an IRB reviewed protocol. However, complementary techniques such as acupuncture may be used at the discretion of the provider and patient.

Recommendations:

1. Complementary-alternative medicine treatments may be considered as adjunctive treatments or when requested by individuals with concussion/mTBI. [SR = I]

Annotation B-9 *Follow-Up and Assess in 4-6 Weeks*

6. Follow-Up

Recommendations:

1) All patients should be followed up in 4 – 6 weeks to confirm resolution of symptoms and address any concerns the patient may have.
2) Follow-up after the initial interventions is recommended in all patients to determine patient status. The assessment will determine the following course of treatment:
   a) Patient recovers from acute symptoms – provide contact information with instructions for available follow-up if needed.
   b) Patient demonstrates partial improvement (e.g., less frequent headaches, resolution of physical symptoms, but no improvement in sleep) – consider augmentation or adjustment of the current intervention and follow-up within 4-6 weeks.
   c) Patient does not improve or status worsens – Focus should be given to other factors including psychiatric, psychosocial support, and compensatory/litigation. Referral to a specialty provider should be considered.

C: Follow-up Management of Persistent Concussion/mTBI Symptoms

Annotation C-1 Person Diagnosed with Concussion/mTBI and Persistent Symptoms Beyond 4-6 Weeks

The vast majority of individuals with concussion/mTBI will have no difficulties or complaints following injury.

While early interventions have been shown to prevent physical, cognitive and behavioral deficits, certain individuals will have persistent difficulties.

Additionally, a significant percentage of individuals with concussion/mTBI will not receive early diagnosis or will not seek treatment, and therefore their symptoms will be addressed only after a temporal delay. This guideline recommends that these individuals should first be treated following the algorithm and annotations in the sections addressing initial presentation and diagnosis.

For patients with symptoms that do not respond to initial treatment, the recommendations in this section will apply. This section also includes suggestions for further evaluations and for referrals to specialty providers.

Annotation C-2 Reassess Symptom Severity and Functional Status Complete Psychosocial Evaluation

7. Assessment of Persistent Symptoms

Background: In patients with persistent post-concussive symptoms that have been refractory to treatment, consideration should be given to other factors, including behavioral health (e.g., stress disorders, mood disorders, and substance use disorders), psychosocial support, and compensation/litigation.

Recommendations:

1) Follow-up after the initial interventions is recommended in all patients with concussion/mTBI to determine patient status and the course of treatment.
2) Evaluation of patients with persistent symptoms following concussion/mTBI should include assessment for dangerousness to self or others.
3) In assessment of patients with persistent symptoms, focus should be given to other factors including psychiatric, psychosocial support, and compensation/litigation issues and a comprehensive psychosocial evaluation should be obtained, to include:
    a) Support systems (e.g., family, vocational)
    b) Mental health history for pre-morbid conditions which may impact current care
    c) Co-occurring conditions (e.g., chronic pain, mood disorders, stress disorder, personality disorder)
    d) Substance use disorder (e.g., alcohol, prescription misuse, illicit drugs, caffeine)
    e) Secondary gain issues (e.g., compensation, litigation)
    f) Unemployment or/change in job status
    g) Other issues (e.g., financial/housing/legal).

Discussion:

Table C-1 includes key domains of functional assessment and suggested questions to guide the patient assessment.

7.1. Risk Factors for Persistent Post-Concussion Symptoms

Background: Identifying risk factors for persisting symptoms and understanding the relationship between risk factors and short- and long-term outcomes can help enhance assessment and treatment.

Some risks are pre-existing factors that may predispose an individual to worse outcomes following a concussion/mTBI; others are potentially directly causative (e.g., the injury itself or medical/legal iatrogenic factors); and still others are potentially perpetuating factors which may occur during the peri-injury or post-injury timeframe.

Recommendations:

1. Assessment of the patient with concussion/mTBI should include a detailed history regarding potential pre-injury, peri-injury, or post-injury risk factors for poorer outcomes. These risk factors include:

a) *Pre-injury:* older age, female gender, low socio-economic status, low education or lower levels of intellectual functioning, poorer coping abilities or less resiliency, pre-existing mental health conditions (e.g., depression, anxiety, PTSD, substance use disorders).

b) *Peri-injury:* lower levels of or less available social support
c) *Post-injury:* injury-related litigation or compensation, comorbid mental health conditions or chronic pain, lower levels of or less available social support,

2. Any substance abuse and/or intoxication at the time of injury should be documented.
3. Establish and document if the patient with concussion/mTBI experienced headaches, dizziness, or nausea in the hours immediately following the injury.

Table C-1. Functional Assessment

Work	• Have there been any changes in productivity? • Have co-workers or supervisors commented on any recent changes in appearance, quality of work, or relationships? • Is there an increase in tardiness, loss of motivation, or loss of interest? • Has the patient been more forgetful, easily distracted?
School	• Have there been changes in grades? • Have there been changes in relationships with friends? • Has there been a recent onset or increase in acting-out behaviors? • Has there been a recent increase in disciplinary actions? • Has there been increased social withdrawal? • Has there been a change in effort required to complete assignments?
Family Relationships	• Have there been negative changes in relationship with significant others? • Is the patient irritable or easily angered by family members? • Has there been a withdrawal of interest in or time spent with family? • Has there been any violence within the family?
Housing	• Does the patient have adequate housing? • Are there appropriate utilities and services? • Is the housing situation stable?
Legal	• Are there outstanding warrants, restraining orders, or disciplinary actions? • Is the person regularly engaging in, or at risk to be involved in, illegal activity? • Is the patient on probation or parole? • Is the patient seeking litigation for compensation? • Is there family advocacy/Department of Social Services (DSS) involvement?
Financial	• Does the patient have the funds for current necessities including food, clothing, and shelter? • Is there a stable source of income? • Are there significant outstanding or past-due debts, alimony, child support? • Has the patient filed for bankruptcy? • Does the patient have access to healthcare and/or insurance?
Unit/ Community Involvement	• Does the patient need to be put on profile, MEB, or limited duty? • Is the patient functional and contributing in the unit environment? • Is there active/satisfying involvement in a community group or organization?

Annotation C-3 Assess for Possible Alternative Causes for Persistent Symptoms

Table C-2. Risk Factors for Persistent Symptoms and/or Poorer Overall Outcomes

Pre-injury	Peri-injury	Post-injury
- Age (older)	**- Lack of support system**	**- Compensation**
- Gender (female)	- Acute symptom presentation(e.g., headaches, dizziness, or nausea in the ER)	**- Litigation (malingering, delayed** resolution)
- Low SES		
- Less education / Lower levels of intelligence		**- Co-occurrence of psychiatric disorders**
- Pre-neurological conditions	- Context of injury (stress, combat-related, traumatic)	- Co-occurrence of chronic pain conditions
- Pre- or co-occurrence of mental health disorders (depression, anxiety, traumatic stress, or substance use)		- Lack of support system **- Low education**

Bold text indicates support of Level C evidence.

Evidence Statements:

Previous Head Injury

- History of prior head injury has been shown to be associated with poorer outcomes in terms of lingering symptoms (Binder, 1997; Ponsford et al., 2000).

Demographic

- There is consistent evidence that older age individuals who sustain a concussion/mTBI have poorer outcomes in terms of sustained symptoms (Binder, 1997; McCauley, 2001; Farace and Alves, 2000).
- Well-designed observational studies indicate that females have increased risk of developing post-concussive symptoms following mTBI (Binder, 1997; Bazarian et al., 2001; Broshek et al., 2005; McCauley, 2001).
- Lower levels of education or IQ are associated with greater levels or duration of post-concussion symptoms (Binder, 1997; Colligan et al., 2005; Dawson et al., 2007; Luis et al., 2003).

Social Support

- Lower level of social support or higher level of psychosocial stress are risk factors for longterm post-concussive symptoms (Luis et al., 2003; McCauley, 2001).

Mental Health

- Individuals with pre-existing mental health problems are more likely to have sustained post-concussion symptoms (Binder, 1997; Evered et al., 2003; Luis et al., 2003, Kashluba et al., 2008).
- Co-morbid mental health problems are associated with higher levels or greater duration of post-concussion symptoms (Colligan et al., 2005; Ponsford et al., 2000).
- The prevalence of chronic pain was greater in patients with mTBI than with moderate or severe TBI. Chronic pain contributes to morbidity and poor recovery after brain injury. (Nampiaparampil, 2008).
- There are contradictory findings on whether substance abuse and/or intoxication at the time of injury is associated with poorer outcomes (Ashman et al., 2004; Bigler et

al., 1996; Bombardier et al., 2003; MacMillan et al., 2002) or not (Dikmen et al., 2004, Moldover et al., 2004; Turner et al., 2006).

Peri-Injury Factors

- Peri-injury severity variables within the criteria of mTBI, including GCS, duration of PTA, and presence of loss of consciousness (LOC), *have not been* shown to be an independent predictor of persistent long-term symptoms (Carroll et al., 2004; Dawson et al., 2007; Iverson et al., 2006; van der Naalt et al., 2001).
- Substance abuse and/or intoxication at the time of injury may be associated with poorer psychological and functional outcomes (Ashman et al., 2004; Bigler et al., 1996; Bombardier et al., 2003; Colligan, et al., 2005; MacMillan et al., 2002) but others have not found this relationship (Dikmen et al., 2004; Moldover et al., 2004; Turner et al., 2006).
- Early symptoms of headaches, dizziness, or nausea in the immediate period (e.g., in the Emergency Department) after mTBI have been associated with sustained post-concussion symptoms months after injury (Chamelian & Feinstein, 2004; de Kruijk et al., 2002).

Post-Injury Litigation/Compensation

- Litigation or compensation seeking at time of assessment has consistently been associated with greater levels of symptoms and poorer outcomes (Binder & Rohling, 1996; Carroll et al., 2004; Suhr et al., 1997, Kashluba et al., 2008).

7.2. Compensation Seeking/Non-Validated Symptoms

Background: The majority of people with concussion/mTBI will have no difficulties or complaints following injury. However, a minority of patients will continue to have ongoing symptoms that may result in a disability. Though these symptoms lose specificity with time and may be wrongly attributed to the mTBI/concussion, they may also interfere with an individual's recovery. Even after a careful differential diagnosis, it remains a challenge for providers to quantify non-specific, subjective complaints for the purposes of disability compensation.

Recommendations:

1. Symptom exaggeration or compensation seeking should not influence the clinical care rendered, and doing so can be counter-therapeutic and negatively impact the quality of care.
2. Focus of the provider-patient interaction should be on the development of a therapeutic alliance (SR=C).

Evidence Statements: Although there is compelling evidence of a relationship between persistence of symptoms and litigation/compensation seeking, this relationship is complex, and there is no therapeutic benefit to attributing symptom expression to malingering or intentional efforts to receive compensation.

- Multiple researchers have found that there is compelling evidence that individuals in litigation or seeking compensation following concussion/mTBI have poorer long-term outcomes. Binder & Rohlings (1996), in a meta-analysis looking at the effect of money on recovery after mTBI, recommended that clinicians consider the effects of financial incentives.

- There is compelling evidence that individuals in litigation or seeking compensation following mTBI have poorer long-term outcomes, including requiring more days to return to work (Gottshall et al., 2007; Reynolds, 2003), greater symptom severity (Paniak et al., 2002) and poorer neuropsychological functioning (Belanger et al., 2005a).
- There is also some evidence to suggest that compensation-seeking behavior resolves more rapidly with immediate compensation, such as sick pay and/or worker's compensation (Reynolds et al., 2003; Rose et al., 2005).
- There is evidence to support the conclusion that non-validated symptoms occur with higher frequency in individuals with mTBI who are seeking compensation and that the incidence of such symptoms increases with higher financial incentives (Bianchini, et al., 2006).

7.3. Persistent Post-Concussive Symptoms (PPCS)

Background: For concussion/mTBI patients, most symptoms and signs that occur in the acute period resolve quickly (within hours or days) after the injury. There is debate about the incidence of developing persistent symptoms after concussion, largely due to the lack of an accepted case definition for persistent symptoms and the fact that none of the symptoms are specific to concussion. There is no consensus on a case definition for persistent symptoms attributed to concussion/mTBI and no consensus on the time course when acute symptoms should be considered persistent.

See discussion in Section 1.6 Persistent Symptoms after Concussion, and Table C-3 Post-Concussion Symptoms.

Table C-3. Post-Concussion Symptoms

Somatic Symptoms	Psychological	Cognitive
• Headache *	• Problems controlling emotions *	• Problems with memory *
• Fatigue *		• Cognitive disorders *
• Sensitivity to light/noise *	• Irritability *	• Problems with concentration *
• Insomnia & sleep disturbances *	• Anxiety *	• Functional status limitations *
• Drowsiness * • Dizziness * • Nausea & vomiting * • Vision problems * • Transient neurological abnormalities • Seizures • Balance problems	• Depression *	

* In common with Post Concussive Syndrome (PCS)

Recommendations:

1. For clinical treatment purposes the use of post-concussion syndrome, post-concussive syndrome (PCS) or post-concussion disorder (PCD) as a diagnosis is not recommended. The unique individual pattern of symptoms should be documented and be the focus of treatment.

For the purpose of this CPG, the term *persistent post-concussive symptoms* will be used.

Discussion: Somatic, cognitive and behavioral symptoms after concussion/mTBI rapidly resolve by 2 to 4 weeks in the majority individuals (McCrea, 2003).

The term *post-concussion syndrome* (PCS), also known as *post-concussive syndrome* (PCS) or *post-concussion disorder* (PCD) is used for individuals who have persistent non-focal, neurologic symptoms (at least 2), most commonly dizziness, headache, cognitive deficits (attention, memory, and judgment), behavioral changes (irritability, depression, nightmares) and/or sleep disturbance.

- In late or persistent PCS, symptoms last for over six months.
- The PCS cluster of symptoms is not unique to concussion (occurs with many medical and psychiatric conditions as well as in normal individuals)
- The exact cluster of symptoms varies substantially across concussion patients; therefore it does not meet criteria for a "syndrome."
- The definition of PCS is plagued by several factors including poor reliability of diagnostic criteria and no specificity of PCS symptoms.
- PCS is seen in between 15% (DSM-IV) to 50% (WHO-ICD-10) of persons with mTBI, depending on how it is defined (McCrea, 2003).
- For all individuals with an initial mTBI, <5% may have persistent difficulties by 12 months (Iverson, 2007).
- Physical symptoms dominate in the first 4 weeks after injury, whereas emotional disturbances predominate later (at 4 - 8 weeks) (Yang, 2007).

Annotation C-4 Any Behavioral Health Diagnosis Established?

7.4. Persistent Behavioral Symptoms

Background: Patients with persistent post-concussive symptoms have a higher incidence of co-occurring mental health conditions (e.g., Stress disorders [ASD, PTSD]), other anxiety disorders, mood disorders, Substance Use Disorders [SUD]) and a pre-injury history of mental health conditions.

In patients with persistent post-concussive symptoms (PPCS), that have been refractory to treatment, a referral to mental health may help elucidate other factors which may be involved in the exacerbation or maintenance of concussion symptoms. These include prior psychiatric history, lack of psychosocial support, financial compensation/litigation, chronic pain, and somatoform spectrum disorders.

See Table C-6: Behavioral Symptoms – TREATMENT

Recommendations:

1) Patients with persistent symptoms following concussion/mTBI should be re-evaluated for psychiatric symptoms and co-morbid psychiatric disorders.
2) Treatment of psychiatric symptoms following concussion/mTBI beyond the acute phase should still be based on individual factors and nature and severity of symptom presentation, including psychotherapeutic [SR = A] and pharmacologic [SR = I] treatment modalities.
3) In patients with persistent post- concussive symptoms (PPCS), which have been refractory to treatment, consideration should be given to other factors including psychiatric disorders, lack of psychosocial support, and compensation/litigation.

Annotation C-5 Consider Referral to Specialty Care

8. Consultation And Referral

Recommendations:

1. A consultation or referral to specialists should occur in a patient with concussion/mTBI who complains of persistent or chronic symptoms when:

a) An atypical pattern or course (worsening or variable symptom presentation) is demonstrated
b) The patient is experiencing difficulties in return to pre-injury activity (work/duty/school)
c) Problems emerge in the role of the patient in family or social life.

2. Patients with multiple problems may benefit from an inter-disciplinary approach to include occupational therapy, recreation therapy, social work, psychology and/or psychiatry, neurology, ENT, ophthalmology or audiology, based on individual symptoms. The patient's provider should remain involved in the patient's care.

3. Referral to mental health specialty of patients with persistent behavioral symptoms should be considered.

See Table C-4 Indications for Referral to Mental Health

7.5. Persistent Physical Symptoms

Recommendations:

1. Patients who are refractory to treatment of physical symptoms in the initial care setting should be referred to specialty care for further evaluation and management (**See** Appendix D – Treatment of Physical Symptoms).

See Table C-5 Physical Symptoms – TREATMENT

7.6. Persistent Cognitive Difficulties

Background: Although initial cognitive complaints and problems are common in the first hours and days after a concussion/mTBI, the vast majority of individuals recover within one to four weeks.

However, a small minority either continue to report cognitive problems or report worsening symptoms over the months and even years post-injury.

This subgroup frequently has premorbid or comorbid conditions such as depression, anxiety, poor health, and chronic pain or poor psychosocial support or other coping resources.

Assistive technology for cognition (ATC) refers to a subset of assistive technology used to compensate for cognitive impairments in memory, attention, and executive function.

Table C-4. Indications for Referral to Mental Health

- Failure to respond to acute supportive interventions
- Worsening of stress related symptoms
- High potential for dangerousness
- Development of PTSD
- Exacerbation of pre-existing psychiatric conditions
- Deterioration in function
- New onset stressors, poor social supports or inadequate coping skills
- Impairment in family or vocational role function

Annotation C-6 Any Persistent Symptoms (Physical, Cognitive or Emotional)?

Devices in this category are also known as memory aids or cognitive prostheses. They are designed to assist individuals with concussion/mTBI to carry out everyday tasks by providing cues or limiting demands on impaired cognitive skills.

Devices can range from simple electronic tools, such as a wrist watch with an alarm function to sophisticated personal digital assistants and global positioning systems. Successful long-term utilization of ATC by persons with concussion/mTBI requires selection of appropriate devices and effective training using the device in real-life contexts.

See Table C-6 Cognitive Symptoms – TREATMENT

Recommendations:

1) Patients who have cognitive symptoms that do not resolve or have been refractory to treatment should be considered for referral for neuropsychological assessment.
   The evaluation may assist in clarifying appropriate treatment options based on individual patient characteristics and conditions. [SR = B]
2) Neuropsychological testing should only be conducted with reliable and standardized tools by trained evaluators, under controlled conditions, and findings interpreted by trained clinicians. [SR = C]
3) Individuals who present with memory, attention, and/or executive function problems which did not respond to initial treatment (e.g., reassurance, sleep education, or pain management) may be considered for referral to cognitive rehabilitation therapists with expertise in TBI rehabilitation (e.g., speech and language pathology, neuropsychology, or occupational therapy) for compensatory training [SR = C]; and/or instruction and practice on use of external memory aids such as a PDA. [SR = C]

Evidence Statements:

- Some studies show that a subgroup of individuals continue to have both subjective symptoms (Alves et al., 1993; Deb et al., 1999; Dikmen et al., 1986; Hartlage et al., 2001; Luis et al., 2003; Powell et al., 1996) and lower cognitive test performance even after 90 days (Belanger et al., 2005; Binder et al., 1997; Vanderploeg et al., 2005)
- There is limited support for the effect of working memory and dual task training on improving attention and processing speed following in mild TBI (Cicerone et al., 2002).
- One study found that even in the chronic phase a combination of psychotherapy, support, and cognitive remediation treatment improved symptoms and actual cognitive performance (Tiersky et al., 2005).
- A systematic review of the literature in the moderate to severe TBI rehabilitation literature showed that attention, memory, and executive functioning deficits after TBI can be improved using interventions emphasizing strategy training (i.e., training patients to compensate for residual deficits, rather than attempting to eliminate the underlying neurocognitive impairment) including use of assistive technology or memory aids (Cicerone et al., 2005).

Table C-5. Persistent Physical Symptoms – TREATMENT

Common Symptoms Following concussion/mTBI	Pharmacologic Treatment	Non-Pharmacologic Treatment	Referral After Failed Response to Initial Treatment
Headaches	-Non narcotic pain meds -NSAIDs -Triptans (migraine type)	-Sleep education -Physical therapy -Relaxation	Neurology Pain clinic
Feeling dizzy	-Antibiotics, decongestants for infections and fluid	-	Dizzy : ENT/Neurology after ENT interventions
Loss of balance Poor coordination	-	-Physical therapy	Neurology
Nausea	-Antiemetics	-Sleep education	GI
Change in appetite	-	-	Consider Mental Health
Sleep disturbances - Difficulty falling or staying asleep (insomnia)	-Sleep Medications	-Sleep education	Mental health PM&R Neurology
Vision problems - Blurring - Trouble seeing - Sensitivity to light	-	-Sleep education -Light desensitization -Sunglasses	Optometry Ophthalmology **
Hearing difficulty - Sensitivity to noise	-	-Environmental modifications	Audiology ENT Sensitivity to Noise : Speech and Language Pathology

Depending on the local resources, impaired vision may be referred in some facilities to neuro-ophthalmologists. Note that the impaired vision may be due to problems with oculomotility as well as due to disorders of the retina and visual pathways.

Table C-6. Persistent Behavioral and Cognitive Symptoms – TREATMENT

<table>
<tr><th>Common Symptoms Following Concussion/mTBI</th><th>Job Review</th><th>Pharmacologic Treatment</th><th>Non-Pharmacologic Treatment</th><th>Referral after failed response to initial intervention</th></tr>
<tr><td>Fatigue
- Loss of energy
- Getting tired easily</td><td>√</td><td>Stimulant*</td><td rowspan="4">Reassurance

Encourage regular scheduled aerobic exercise

Activity restriction adjustment

Sleep hygiene Education
Sleep study</td><td>- Mental Health</td></tr>
<tr><td>Cognitive difficulties - Concentration - Memory
- Decision-making</td><td></td><td>SSRI Stimulant*</td><td>- TBI specialist for cognitive rehabilitation or mental health</td></tr>
<tr><td>Feeling anxious</td><td>√</td><td>Anxiolytic (short term)
SSRI</td><td rowspan="2">- Mental Health -
Social support</td></tr>
<tr><td>Emotional difficulties
- Feeling depressed
- Irritability
- Poor frustration tolerance</td><td></td><td>Anti epileptics SSRI</td></tr>
</table>

* Consider in the specialty care setting after ruling out a sleep disorder.

Annotation C-7 *Consider Referral to Occupational or Vocational Therapy and Community Integration Programs (Continue Case Management)*

9. Rehabilitation of Patients with Persistent Post-Concussion Symptoms (PPCS)

Background:

Role of Consultants: For patients who will be referred to specialty care, treatment will be provided by the specialty consultant as recommended in the management of specific symptoms or other clinical practice guidelines. The referring care provider is expected to serve as the focal point for an inter-disciplinary approach to treatment that may span the continuum of care. With patient consent, it may be found useful to involve the patient's employer/supervisor, spouse, and friends and significant others within the patient's social support network.

In patients with persistent post concussion/mTBI symptoms (PPCS), the role of mental health providers (psychiatry, psychology, neuropsychology, social work, and others) will be more essential in providing input into implementing psychotherapeutic treatment in the outpatient setting. Social workers should help build family and social support networks, or recommend changes in the patient's living situation, in order to create a positive support network.

9.1. Case Management in the Care of Patients with mTBI

Background: Patients presenting with symptoms should be considered both initially and on an ongoing basis for referral to case management. Whether the patient has recently returned from deployment or combat, or is a veteran who has sustained non-combat related head trauma, the need for a collaborative and coordinated approach to comprehensive care is necessary.

Table C-7. Case Managers Serve Multiple Functions

- Complete an in-depth assessment of functional status and coordinate treatment resources
- Ensure that the patient is screened for social service needs and mental health problems.
- Assure that referrals are coordinated and made as appropriate to the responsible discipline
- Ensure that the patient and family have received appropriate education
- Participate in setting short- and long-term goals
- Assist in the process of moving between facilities and levels of care
- Monitor patient progress
- Coordinate and collaborate with the multi-disciplinary team

Recommendations:

1) Patients with persistent symptoms following concussion/mTBI may be considered for case management.
2) Case managers should complete a comprehensive psychosocial assessment of the patient and the patient's family.
   It may be necessary or beneficial to meet with other members of the patient's support system (family, care giver) and/or invite the patient to ask them to come to an appointment together with the patient.
3) Case managers should collaborate with the treatment team, the patient, and the patient's family in developing a treatment plan that emphasizes the psychosocial needs of the patient.
4) Case managers (in collaboration with the treatment team) should prepare and document a detailed treatment plan in the medical record describing follow-up care and services required.
5) Case managers who provide care in the clinical setting should communicate and coordinate with other potential care coordinators that provide care for the patient (such as a VHA social worker liaison or military social worker at the referring Military Treatment Facility, Patient Treatment Advocate (PTA)).
6) Case managers may provide assistance to the patient and family who are transferred to another facility (e.g., a polytrauma rehabilitation center).
7) Case management may serve as the main point of contact for the patient and family. This may include the following:
   a) Provide the patient with contact information including after hours calls
   b) Maintain frequent contact by phone to remind about or facilitate an appointment
   c) Facilitate access to supportive services to the patient and family
   d) Serve as a liaison for the patient's family and as an advocate for the patient and the patient's family

e) Provide easy-to-understand information in writing for the patient and the patient's family.

9.2. Patient and Family Education

Recommendations:

1) All members of the treatment team should be involved in patient education as part of their interaction with the patient experiencing persistent symptoms.
2) Educational interventions should generally include information and a description of the specific procedures and events the patient will experience at the various phases of treatment and continue throughout the continuum of care.
3) General supportive counseling (e.g., eliciting and validating the patient's anxieties, fears, and concerns) may also be helpful. Open-ended questioning, active listening techniques, eliciting anticipation of future stressors, encouraging the patient to ask questions, and eliciting and encouraging utilization of the patient's social support resources are important strategies regardless of whether information-giving or coping skills training interventions are being used.
4) Educational interventions may also include coping techniques for symptom management, such as patient education handouts and helpful tips.

See Appendix B: Health Risk Communication

9.3. Functional and Vocational Activities

Background:

A return to the normal patterns of daily life and safe, independent living requires a practical, individualized application of therapeutically-based treatment. This includes the assessment and reestablishment of structured routines in daily activities, marriage/family dynamics, educational activities, vocation, and community involvement. The emphasis of the team at this point is to enhance functional outcome and reduce disability associated with the symptoms. This is accomplished by treatment that improves patient function and by interventions that mitigate and adjust the environment in which the patient is expected to function (e.g., family, vocational and community). Potentially modifiable psychosocial barriers to patient functioning could include the following:

- **Living environment**—Homelessness can perpetuate chronic illness as the result of environmental exposure and virtually non-existent personal hygiene.
- **Support systems**—Negative supports on the part of the spouse, family, or significant other can impair and even worsen functionality.
- **Job**—Work place factors have been associated with illness-related behavior.
- **Finances**—Disability compensation can perpetuate illness by requiring continuing symptoms and disability for the worker to be eligible for benefits.

Recommendations:

Family Support

1) As with other chronic conditions, the focus of the management of patients with persistent symptoms following concussion/mTBI should shift to the psychological and social impacts on the patient.

2) The clinician should consider having the spouse or partner accompany the patient with concussion/mTBI to a consultation, to help them better understand the condition and provide an opportunity to discuss any coping difficulties.
3) Family members should be encouraged to consider joining a support group to provide education, advice and opportunities to exchange coping strategies for dealing with the day-to-day difficulties of living with an individual with persistent symptoms following concussion/mTBI.

Vocational Rehabilitation

1. Vocational interventions for the patient with persistent symptoms following concussion/mTBI may include modifications such as:

- Modification of the length of the work day
- Gradual work re-entry (e.g., starting at 2 days/week and expanding to 3 days/week)
- Additional time for task completion
- Change of job
- Environmental modifications (e.g., quieter work environment; enhanced level of supervision)

2. Patients who have not successfully resumed pre-injury work duties following injury should be referred for a vocational evaluation by clinical specialists with expertise in assessing and treating concussion/mTBI.

3. For patients with persistent symptoms following concussion/mTBI, return to full work/duty in the jobs they have previously preformed may not be possible. Patients may need to proceed through medical or disability evaluation processes.

This process should follow national and local regulations and is beyond the scope of the guideline.

Community Participation:

4. A referral to a structured program that promotes community integration may be considered for individuals with residual persistent post-concussive symptoms that impede return to pre-injury participation in customary roles.

Discussion: *Vocational Rehabilitation:* Following a concussion/mTBI, most individuals are able to resume normal work duties within a week to month with secondary prevention precautions and education requiring little or no additional therapeutic intervention.

A small percentage of individuals with concussion/mTBI may be instructed to temporarily reduce the amount, type and/or intensity of their work duties or temporarily remain out of work entirely.

In instances where residual impairments are such that a career change may be needed, referral to a vocational rehabilitation program that provides comprehensive services, e.g., assessment, identification of work skills, alternatives for future employment, and referral for training and education may be considered.

Clinicians may be asked to act as advocates for their patients in negotiations with employers, educational institutions, and social welfare organizations. For instance, the patient may need assistance in arranging part-time work or school alternatives or securing disability allowances.

In a survey of concussion/mTBI patients 4 to 6 months post-injury, key emerging issues for participants who return to work were the invisibility of their injury, continuing symptoms affecting their ability to do their job and lack of advice and guidance on returning to work. Return to work support systems were considered to be poorly coordinated and managed (Gilworth et al., 2008).

Community Participation (also called Community Reintegration): This refers to the resumption of age, gender, and culturally appropriate roles in the family, community and workplace.

Individuals with residual symptoms from concussion/mTBI experiencing problems returning to their pre-injury level of activity may benefit from individual and/or group interventions that focus on development of skills and strategies to address impairments (e.g., behavior regulation, interpersonal relationships, and functional cognition). Cicerone (2005) suggests that intensive cognitive rehabilitation seems to help with community integration in individuals with moderate to severe TBI.

Additionally, it appears that peer support groups result in higher reported quality of life scores and less depressive symptoms (Hibbard, 2002).

Annotation C- 8 *Follow-Up and Reassess in 3-4 Months*

10. Follow-up

Background: The goal of follow-up visits is to monitor the severity of symptoms, impact of the symptoms on activities, effects of treatments, and presence of adverse effects to treatments, and to assess patients for new symptoms suggestive of other diagnoses.

Although natural improvement is generally expected, recovery can be prolonged and a minority of patients still have symptoms at 6 months. The use of telephonic and other distance technologies may be used to monitor the recovery process, reinforce education, and prevent development of secondary problems.

Recommendations:

1. Scheduled follow-up visits are recommended. The amount of time between visits will vary depending on a number of factors, including the following:

a. Quality of the provider/patient relationship

- Distress of the patient
- Need for refinement of the treatment plan or additional support – Presence or absence of psychosocial stressors.

b. Severity of the symptoms

- Initially, a follow-up at two to three weeks would be appropriate
- As soon as the patient is doing well, then follow-up every 3 to 4 months would be recommended
- Telephone follow-up may be sufficient to evaluate resolution of symptoms and reinforce education.

c. For concussion/mTBI patients with complicated histories, comorbidities, and lack of social support consider case management.

2. Continually re-evaluate the patient for worsening of chronic symptoms or presence of new symptoms suggestive of other diagnoses.

APPENDICES

Appendix A: Guideline Development Process

The development of the VA/DoD Clinical Practice Guideline for Management of Concussion/mTBI followed the steps described in "Guideline for Guidelines," an internal working document of the VA/DoD Evidence Based Practice Working Group, that requires an ongoing review of the work in progress. The Working Group of the VA/DoD was charged to update the evidence-based action recommendations whenever possible.

The Offices of Quality and Performance and Patient Care Services, in collaboration with the network Clinical Managers, the Deputy Assistant Under Secretary for Health, and the U.S. Army Medical Command for the DoD identified clinical leaders to champion the guideline development process. During a preplanning conference call, the clinical leaders defined the scope of the guideline and identified a group of clinical experts from the VA and DoD that formed the Management of Concussion/mTBI Working Group. Working Group members included representatives of the following specialties: primary care, internal medicine, physical medicine and rehabilitation (PM&R), psychiatry, neuropsychology, neurology, neurophysiology, neuroradiology, social work/case management, occupational therapy, physical therapy, speech-language therapy, and vocational therapy.

The Working Group defined a set of clinical questions within the area of the guideline. This ensured that the guideline development work outside the meeting focused on issues that practitioners considered important and produced criteria for the search and the protocol for systematic review and, where appropriate, meta-analysis.

The Working Group participated in an initial face-to-face meeting to reach consensus about the guideline algorithm and recommendations and to prepare a draft update document. The draft continued to be revised by the Working Group at-large through numerous conference calls and individual contributions to the document. Following the initial effort, an editorial panel of the Working Group convened to further edit the draft document. Recommendations for the performance or inclusion of specific procedures or services were derived through a rigorous methodological approach that included the following:

- Determining appropriate criteria, such as effectiveness, efficacy, population benefit, or patient satisfaction
- Reviewing literature to determine the strength of the evidence in relation to these criteria
- Formulating the recommendations and grading the level of evidence supporting the recommendation

- Experts from the VA and DoD reviewed the final draft and their feedback was integrated into the final draft document.

This update of the Concussion/mTBI Guideline is the product of many months of diligent effort and consensus building among knowledgeable individuals from the VA, DoD, academia, as well as guideline facilitators from the private sector. An experienced moderator facilitated the multidisciplinary Working Group. The list of participants is included in Appendix H.

Formulation of Questions: The Working Group developed researchable questions and associated key terms after orientation to the scope of the guideline and to goals that had been identified by the Working Group. The questions specified:

- Population – Characteristics of the target patient population
- Intervention – Exposure, diagnostic, or prognosis
- Comparison – Intervention, exposure, or control used for comparison
- Outcome – Outcomes of interest.

These specifications served as the preliminary criteria for selecting studies. Literature searches were conducted on all topics identified in the algorithm or recommendations. After reviewing the initial search for systematic reviews and meta-analyses, the Working Group decided to focus the search for individual randomized controlled trials (RCT) on the following questions:

Questions for Literature Search

1) Is there a difference in intervention in individuals with repeated concussion or repeated mTBI?
2) Is there a relationship between self-awareness and response to treatment of cognitive and psychological deficits in individuals with mTBI?
3) Do educational interventions decrease the incidence & severity of chronic mTBI symptoms and lead to better outcomes in individuals with mTBI-related symptoms.
4) Do early cognitive-behavioral interventions decrease the incidence & severity of chronic mTBI symptoms and lead to better outcomes in individuals with mTBI-related symptoms?
5) Are there compensatory strategies/techniques that have been shown to result in better outcomes in individuals with mTBI?
6) Do treatment techniques for vestibular disorders (liberatory maneuvers, balance exercises, computerized posturography) reduce symptoms and provide long-term improvement in outcome in patients with mTBI?

Selection of Evidence: The evidence selection was designed to identify the best available evidence to address each key question and ensure maximum coverage of studies at the top of the hierarchy of study types. Published, peer-reviewed RCTs, as well as meta-analyses and systematic reviews that included randomized controlled studies were considered to constitute the strongest level of evidence in support of guideline recommendations. This decision was based on the judgment that RCTs provide the clearest, most scientifically sound basis for judging comparative efficacy. The Working Group made this decision recognizing the limitations of RCTs, particularly considerations of generalizability with respect to patient selection and treatment quality. When available, the search sought out critical appraisals already performed by others that described explicit criteria for deciding what evidence was selected and how it was determined to be valid. The sources that have already undergone rigorous critical appraisal include Cochrane Reviews, Best Evidence, Technology Assessment, and AHRQ systematic evidence reports.

In addition to Medline/PubMed, the following databases were searched: Database of Abstracts of Reviews of Effectiveness (DARE) and Cochrane Central Register of Controlled Trials. For Medline/PubMed searches, limits were set for language (English), and type of research (RCT, systematic reviews and meta-analysis).

As a result of the literature reviews, articles were identified for possible inclusion. These articles formed the basis for formulating the guideline recommendations. The following inclusion criteria were used for studies:

- English language only of studies performed in United States, United Kingdom, Europe, Australia, Japan, New Zealand
- Full articles only
- Study populations age limited to adults greater than 18 years; all races, ethnicities, cultural groups
- Randomized controlled trials or prospective studies
- Published from 2001 to 2008.

Admissible evidence (study design and other criteria):

- Original research studies that provide sufficient detail regarding methods and results to enable use and adjustment of the data and results.
- Randomized controlled trials (RCT); systematic reviews and meta-analyses.
- Relevant outcomes must be able to be abstracted from data presented in the articles.
- Sample sizes must be appropriate for the study question addressed in the paper.

Preparation of Evidence Tables (Reports) and Evidence Rating: The results of the search were organized in evidence summary reports and copies of the original studies were provided to the Working Group for further analysis. Each study was appraised for scientific merit, clinical relevance, and applicability to the populations served by VA and DoD health care system. The body of evidence was rated for quality and level of evidence.

Recommendation and Overall Quality Rating: Evidence-based practice involves integrating clinical expertise with the best available clinical evidence derived from systematic research. The Working Group received an orientation and tutorial on the evidence rating process, reviewed the evidence and independently formulated the Strength of Recommendation (see Table A-1).

Lack of Evidence – Consensus of Experts: Where existing literature was ambiguous or conflicting, or where scientific data was lacking on an issue, recommendations were based on the clinical experience of the Working Group.

Algorithm Format: The goal in developing the guideline for management of Concussion/mTBI was to incorporate the information into a format which would maximally facilitate clinical decision-making.

The use of the algorithm format was chosen because of the evidence that such a format improves data collection, diagnostic and therapeutic decision-making and changes patterns of resource use. However, few guidelines are published in such a format.

Table A-1. Evidence Rating System

A	A strong recommendation that the clinicians provide the intervention to eligible patients. *Good evidence was found that the intervention improves important health outcomes and concludes that benefits substantially outweigh harm.*
B	A recommendation that clinicians provide (the service) to eligible patients. *At least fair evidence was found that the intervention improves health outcomes and concludes that benefits outweigh harm.*
C	No recommendation for or against the routine provision of the intervention is made. *At least fair evidence was found that the intervention can improve health outcomes, but concludes that the balance of benefits and harms is too close to justify a general recommendation.*
D	Recommendation is made against routinely providing the intervention to patients. *At least fair evidence was found that the intervention is ineffective or that harms outweigh benefits.*
I	The conclusion is that the evidence is insufficient to recommend for or against routinely providing the intervention. *Evidence that the intervention is effective is lacking, or poor quality, or conflicting, and the balance of benefits and harms cannot be determined.*

The algorithmic format allows the provider to follow a linear approach to critical information needed at the major decision points in the clinical process, and includes:

- An ordered sequence of steps of care
- Recommended observations
- Decisions to be considered
- Actions to be taken

A clinical algorithm diagrams a guideline into a step-by-step decision tree. Standardized symbols are used to display each step in the algorithm (Society for Medical Decision-Making Committee, 1992).

Arrows connect the numbered boxes indicating the order in which the steps should be followed.

A letter within a box of an algorithm refers the reader to the corresponding annotation. The annotations elaborate on the recommendations and statements that are found within each box of the algorithm.

Included in the annotations are brief discussions that provide the underlying rationale and specific evidence tables. Annotations indicate whether each recommendation is based on scientific data or expert opinion.

A complete bibliography is included in the guideline.

	Rounded rectangles represent a clinical state or condition.
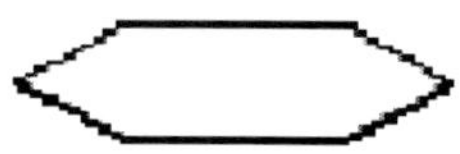	Hexagons represent a decision point in the guideline, formulated as a question that can be answered Yes or No. A horizontal arrow points to the next step if the answer is YES. A vertical arrow continues to the next step for a negative answer.
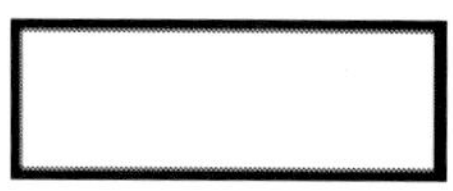	Rectangles represent an action in the process of care.
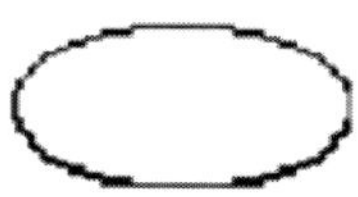	Ovals represent a link to another section within the guideline.

References

Agency for Health Care Policy and Research (AHCPR). Manual for conducting systematic review. *Draft.* August 1996. Prepared by Steven H. Woolf.

Harris RP, Helfand M, Woolf SH, Lohr KN, Mulrow CD, Teutsch SM, Atkins D; Methods Work Group, Third US Preventive Services Task Force Current methods of the U.S. Preventive Services Task Force: a review of the process. *Am J Prev Med 2001* Apr;20(3 Suppl):21-35.

Society for Medical Decision-Making Committee (SMDMC). Proposal for clinical algorithm standards, SMDMC on Standardization of Clinical Algorithms. *Med Decis Making* 1992 Apr-Jun;12(2):149-54.

United States Preventive Service Task Force (USPSTF). Guide to clinical preventive services. 2nd edition. Washington, DC: US Department of Health and Human Services, Office of Disease Prevention and Health Promotion, 1996.

Woolf SH. Practice guidelines, a new reality in medicine II. Methods of developing guidelines. *Arch Intern Med* 1992 May;152(5):946-52.

Appendix B

Structured Interview for Collecting Head Trauma Event Characteristics

Head Trauma Event Characteristics Name: ________________________________ Date/Time of Injury___________________ Reporter: ____ Patient ____ Parent ____Spouse _____ Other	
1	Injury Description 1a. Is there evidence of a forcible blow to the head (direct or indirect)? ____Yes ____ No ____ Unknown
	1b. Is there evidence of intracranial injury or skull fracture? ____ Yes ____ No ____ Unknown
	1c. Location of Impact: ____ Frontal ____ Left temporal ____ Left Parietal ____ Right temporal ____ Right Parietal ____ Occipital ____ Neck ____ Indirect force
2	Cause: ____ MVC ____ Pedestrian-MVC ____ Fall ____ Assault ____ Sports ____ Blast ____ Other (specify) ___________________________
3	Amnesia Before (Retrograde) Are there any events just BEFORE the injury that you/person has no memory of (even brief)? ____ Yes ____ No ____Duration
4	Amnesia After (Anterograde) Are there any events just AFTER the injury that you/person has no memory of (even brief)? ____ Yes ____ No Duration ________
5	Loss of Consciousness Did you/person lose consciousness? ____Yes ____ No Duration _____
6	EARLY SIGNS ___ Appears dazed or stunned ____ Is confused about events ___ Answers questions slowly ____ Repeats Questions ___ Forgetful (recent info)
7	Were seizures observed? ____ No ____Yes Detail ______________
8	Any deaths/injuries to others that occurred as a result of this event? _____ No ____ Yes

Instructions for collecting injury characteristics information

Q1	Obtain description of the injury: how injury occurred, type of force, location on thehead or body (if force transmitted to head). Different biomechanics of injury resultin differential symptom patterns (e.g., occipital blow may result in visual changes, balance difficulties).
Q2	Indicate the cause of injury. Greater forces associated with the trauma are likely to result in more severe presentation of symptoms.
Q3 & 4	Amnesia: Amnesia is defined as the failure to form new memories. Determine whether amnesia has occurred and attempt to determine length of time of memory dysfunction – before (retrograde) and after (anterograde) injury.
Q5	Loss of consciousness (LOC) – If occurs, determine length of LOC.
Q6	Early signs. If present, ask the individuals who know the patient (parent, spouse, friend, etc) about specific signs of the concussion that may have been observed. These signs are typically observed early after the injury.
Q7	Inquire whether seizures were observed or not.
Q8	Deaths or injuries that occur during an event can contribute to the development of mental health symptoms.

Appendix C: Health Risk Communication

Risk communication is the process of exchanging information among interested parties about the nature, magnitude, significance, or control of a risk. [1] In a health care setting, risk communication occurs during every patient visit when discussing diagnoses, medications, treatments or procedures; some topics are more challenging than others. Treating patients with obvious or suspected mTBI/ concussion will likely be complex, due in part to the uncertainty related to the history of the traumatic event; uncertainty related to the exact etiology of the presenting physical symptoms; previous medical treatment provided; the patient's psychosocial, emotional, cognitive, and physical issues; and cultural and/or linguistic issues. In addition, conversations about sensitive issues, such as instances where patients are emotional or when care fails to help the patient, can be very difficult for health care providers and other members of the health care team. Fortunately, research in health communication, particularly in cancer care, has been conducted over the past several decades, providing numerous lessons learned that can be applied to the treatment of mTBI/concussion patients. Patients with good communication skills may have more successful interactions with health care providers; however, this guide is targeted toward the health care provider/ team.

Effective communication is often bypassed in general practice due to time constraints, lack of skills, and priorities. A patient-centered approach that integrates effective risk communication can meet the needs of both patient and health care provider, without sacrificing limited time.[2] Certainly, one of the health care provider's primary tasks is to provide information to the patient, such as treatment plan, possible reasons for symptoms, and medication instructions. But effectively communicating with patients continues to be a source of frustration for many health care providers, particularly under time constraints. While communicating information is important, it is also worth noting that information alone does not necessarily equate to understanding; it is only one component of a doctor-patient partnership deemed to be satisfactory to both parties.

Patients with actual or suspected mTBI/ concussion will likely be emotionally distressed, experiencing anxiety, fear, frustration, confusion, uncertainty, lack of choice and control, helplessness, or hopelessness, and other responses. In primary care settings, 76 percent of patients provided emotional clues, yet health care providers responded positively to these clues only 21 percent of the time.[3] Most health care providers and nurses also incorporate "blocking behaviors" that typically move the discussion away from patient concerns and emotions, [4] yet health care providers who communicate effectively and provide compassionate care have been found to have a positive impact on patients' emotional distress, often in as little as 40 seconds. [5] While many health care providers believe that "patient-centered" visits are more time-consuming, those where the dialogue was primarily psychosocial did not result in visits that were significantly longer than others. [6] Improving risk communication skills can more effectively identify and address patient concerns and emotions without sacrificing time. These skills are especially critical when treating mTBI/ concussion patients where a diagnosis has not yet been established, and cognitive complexity and/or emotional distress may be involved.

Research strongly suggests that the quality of health care provider-patient communications can critically influence the quality of life for patients and families, as well as patient health outcomes. Health care providers understandably rely on a patient's medical information to diagnose and provide treatment; yet clinical care that focuses primarily on biological and physiological factors alone -- if they can even be identified, is likely to be ineffective in relieving symptoms.[7] Improved communications have also been shown to provide benefits to health care providers and health care systems. For example:

- The quality of communications were found to positively affect, in descending order of frequency, emotional health, symptom resolution, function, physiologic measures (i.e., blood pressure), and pain control. [8]
- Improved communications produce more complete information about the patient; align health care provider and patient agendas, using time more wisely; increase patient satisfaction with care provided; increase patient compliance, knowledge, understanding and recall; and ultimately improve the long-term psychologic adjustment of the patient. [9, 10]
- The quality of health communication can influence the physiologic health outcome of diabetic patients, such as blood pressure or blood sugar level. [8]
- Compassionate care has been shown to reduce patients' anxiety and emotional distress.[5]
- Communication that included preparing the cancer patient for diagnosis, giving the patient clear information, providing written information, discussing questions and feelings, and being reassuring may lower anxiety. [11]
- Conversely, reassuring high-anxiety cancer patients before patient's concerns are elicited is not helpful.[12]
- Cancer patients reported greater hope when health care providers actively encourage their participation as partners in determining treatment options. [13]
- Feeling valued, having realistic goals, pain/symptom relief, and meaningful relationships are key factors that increase hope in terminally ill patients. [14]

In order for effective communication to occur, the health care provider-patient relationship must be based on mutual trust. Distrust may be especially acute when a cause or explanation for the patient's concerns has not yet been, or cannot be, readily determined. The effectiveness of communications involving a highly personal issue, such as a patient's individual health, is primarily determined by the patient's perception of trustworthiness and credibility of the health care provider. Trust and credibility may not be quickly or easily established, but can result from building and maintaining partnerships between the health care provider, the patient, and their family over time. Four key factors have been found to influence perceptions of trust and credibility during discussions of high-concern issues: [15]

1) **Caring and empathy**, including perceived sincerity, ability to listen, and to see issues from the perspective of others. Of the four factors, patient perceptions of caring and empathy are the most important.
2) **Competence and expertise**, including perceived intelligence, training, experience, education level, professional attainment, knowledge, and command of information. These are the easiest factors to establish because health care providers are automatically perceived by the public to be credible sources of information.
3) **Dedication and commitment**, including perceived altruism, diligence, self-identification, involvement, and hard work. Perceptions of dedication and

commitment are influenced by patient perceptions of the health care provider's hard work in the pursuit of health goals.
4) **Honesty and openness**, including perceived truthfulness, candidness, fairness, objectivity, and sincerity. Perceptions of this factor result from both nonverbal cues (i.e., posture, eye contact, facial expressions, interruptions, indirect language) and language that convey sincerity and concern. Sensitivity to nonverbal cues is especially invaluable in ultimately understanding and communicating effectively with the patient and their family.

Integrating these factors into a patient-centered approach can better address the needs of both health care provider and patient. Health care providers generally want to provide high-quality clinical care within the time limits provided. But patient expectations of the medical visit, their illness, and the consequences of potential exposures may differ significantly from the health care provider's. Patients bring a set of beliefs about themselves and the meaning of their symptoms and possible injuries to their encounters with the health care provider based on a complex set of factors, to include personal values; perceptions of benefits and level of control; degree of social trust; and heuristics. [16] It is therefore critical for the health care provider and patient to work together collaboratively to set an agenda for each visit, and to develop an appropriate treatment plan.

The goals of the health care provider, therefore, should include attempting to understand the patient's beliefs, informing the patient about pertinent scientific information, and establishing a collaborative and negotiated understanding upon which further communication and work can be based. Excellent risk communication skills are essential in communicating clearly, while effectively addressing the emotional and psychosocial needs of the patients and families. This requires that the health care provider: [17,18,19]

- Build rapport with the patient through compassion and empathy.
- Elicit, acknowledge and discuss the patient's social and emotional concerns.
- Be mindful of the patient's and your own body language.
- Align agendas by exploring the patient's perspective (i.e., what the patient already knows, what the patient wants to know).
- Encourage patient participation in discussions and decision-making; make appropriate adjustments to align expectations, preferences, needs and goals.
- Speak in the patient's language.
- Be completely honest.
- Listen actively by paraphrasing your understanding of patient and family input.
- Convey a sense of optimism and hope regarding diagnosis, treatment, and prognosis.
- Co-create the treatment plan.
- Be prepared for a reaction.

At each patient visit, the health care provider should:

- Ask open-ended questions, focusing on and clarifying psychological issues.
- Ask if there are unaddressed or unresolved concerns.
- Provide orientation statements to help the patient develop appropriate expectations of the visit.

- Speak the patient's language and periodically check for patient understanding, by observing subtle, nonverbal cues of patient confusion; then rephrase or restate the information to validate patient report.
- Be sensitive to nonverbal cues, both your own and those of the patient's.
- Summarize and explain all test results, being sure to address any outstanding or interim test results and consultations that will be reviewed during follow-up visits.
- Offer to include the concerned family member or significant other in follow-up visits, being sensitive to patient preferences.
- Schedule follow-up visits in a timely manner.
- Recognize miscommunications and repair them.

Communicating in a high-concern, low-trust environment, such as when caring for mTBI/concussion patients, can be difficult for even the most skilled health care provider. In order to successfully treat patients with mTBI/ concussion, health care providers and health care systems must support or mandate health risk communication training and patient-centered care and communication. Doing so will help assist in successful information transfer; form more effective health care provider-patient relationships; avoid longer patient visits; and ultimately improve the overall health outcome of patients and families, while limiting caregiver burnout.

References

[1] National Research Council. *Improving Risk Communication.* National Academy Press. Washington, DC. 1989.

[2] Mauksch, LB, Dugdale DC, Dodson, S, et al. Relationship, Communication, and Efficiency in the Medical Encounter. *Archives of Internal Medicine.* July 2008: 168(3): 1387-1395.

[3] Levinson, W, Gorawara-Bhat, R, Lamb, J. A study of patient clues and health care provider responses in primary care and surgical settings. *Journal of the American Medical Association.* August 2000:284(8): 1021-1027.

[4] Beach, WA, Easter, DW, Good, JS, et al. Disclosing and responding to cancer "fears" during oncology interviews. *Social Science and Medicine.* October 2004:60(2005): 893-910.

[5] Fogarty, LA, Curbow, BA, Wingard, JR, et al. Can 40 seconds of compassion reduce patient anxiety? *Journal of Clinical Oncology.* 1999:17(1):371-379.

[6] Roter, DL, Stewart, M, Putnam, SM, et al. Communication Patterns of Primary Care Health care providers. *Journal of the American Medical Association.* 1997:277(4): 350-356.

[7] Wilson IB, Cleary PD. Linking clinical variables with health-related quality of life. A conceptual model of patient outcomes. *Journal of the American Medical Association.* 1995:273:59-65.

[8] Stewart, MA. Effective health care provider-patient communication and health outcomes: A Review. *Canadian Medical Association Journal.* 1995:152(9):1423-1433.

[9] Ray, E. B. *Case Studies in Health Communication*. Lawrence Erlbaum Associates. New Jersey. (1993).

[10] Travaline, JM, Ruchinskas, R, D'Alonzo, GE. Patient-Health care provider Communication: Why and How. *Journal of the American Osteopathic Association*. 2005: 105(1) 13-18.
[11] Schofield, PE, Butow, PN, Thompson, FJ, et al. Psychological responses of patients receiving a diagnosis of cancer. *Annals of Oncology*. 2003:14:48-56.
[12] Stark, D, Kiely, M. Smith, A, et al. Reassurance and the anxious cancer patient. *British Journal of Cancer*. 2004(91):893-899.
[13] Sardell, AN, Trierweiler, SJ. Disclosing the Cancer Diagnosis. *Cancer*. December 1993: 72(11): 3355-3365.
[14] Avery, JA. The "H" in *Hospice* Stands for Hope. *Journal of Advanced Nursing*. 1990: 15: 1250- 1259.
[15] Kolluru, R., Bartell, S., Pitblado, R., et al. "Communicating Risk in Crisis and Non-Crisis Situations." *Risk Management Handbook for Environmental, Health, and Safety Professionals*, Part VI. 1996.
[16] Siegrist, M, Cvetkovich, G. Perception of Hazards: The role of social trust and knowledge. Risk Analysis. 2000:20(5):713-719.
[17] Epstein, RM, Street, RL. *Patient-Centered Communication in Cancer Care: Promoting Healing and Reducing Suffering*. National Cancer Institute, 2007. http://outcomes.cancer.gov/areas/pcc/communication /pcc_monograph.pdf
[18] Tongue, JR, Epps, HR, Forese, LL. Communication Skills for Patient-Centered Care. *Journal of Bone and Joint Surgery*. March 2005: (87-A)3: 652-658.
[19] Back, AL, Arnold, RM, Baile, WF, et al. Approaching Difficult Communication Tasks in Oncology. *Cancer Journal for Health care providers*. 2005: 55: 164-177.

Appendix D. Treatment of Physical Symptoms

This Appendix includes recommendations for treatment of a selected list of physical symptoms that are most common in patients presenting with symptoms following a concussion/mTBI. The recommendations were formulated based on Consensus of clinical experts.

D-1. Headache

Background: Post-traumatic headaches occur acutely in up to 90% of all individuals who sustain a concussion. Post-traumatic headaches usually develop within 7 days of head trauma. The International Headache Society classification category is headaches associated with head and neck trauma.

The category was established because the most frequent forms of civilian head trauma also cause injury to the cervical spinal column, spinal cord and neck musculature. Cervicogenic pain can include headache as well as neck pain. Individuals who sustain head and neck injury can have headaches in which the pain originates from both the head and the neck. Although post-traumatic headaches represent a unique category of headache, they often share features of other types of headaches.

The three most common patterns of post-traumatic headaches are:

1) Tension-type headaches, including cervicogenic component
2) Migraine headaches, or
3) Combined migraine and tension-type headaches.

Recommendations:

ASSESSMENT

Physical Examination

1) Acute assessment focuses on determining if an individual has intracranial pathology as a consequence of the head injury. Include examination of the head and neck; cranial nerve examination including: test of olfaction, funduscopic evaluation, measurement of pupil size and reaction to light, and observation of eye movements. The examination also evaluates muscle strength and tone, gait and upper and lower extremity coordination. Warning signs of intracranial pathology that will require neurosurgical intervention include: drowsiness, impaired motor function (hemiparesis or hemi-ataxia), unsteady gait or inability to stand, vomiting with or without head pain, headache with valsalva maneuvers such as coughing, papilledema or pupil asymmetry of size or reactivity to light. Patients with warning signs of intracranial pathology need to have additional assessment including intracranial imaging.

Table D-1. Criteria for characterizing post-traumatic headaches as tension-like (including cervicogenic) or migraine-like based upon headache features

	Headache Type	
Headache Feature	Tension-like (include cerviogenic pain)	Migraine-like
Pain Intensity	Usually mild-moderate	Often severe or debilitating
Pain Character	Dull, aching, or pressure. Sharp pain may be present, but is not predominant	Throbbing or pulsatile, can also be sharp/stabbing or electric-like
Duration	Usually less than 4 hours	Can last longer than 4 hours
Phono- or photo-phobia	One but not both may be present	One, or both usually present
Able to carry out routine activities /work	Usually	Usually not, or with a decreased level of participation
Location	Bilateral frontal, retro-orbital, temporal, cervical and occipital, or holocephalic	Usually unilateral and may vary in location among episodes
Nausea or malaise	Not present	Usually present
Palpable muscle tenderness or contraction	Pericranial muscles including temporalis, masseter, pterygoid, posterior neck muscle, sternocleidomastoid, splenius or trapezius	Localized muscle tenderness is not typical, muscle tenderness may be present with long duration headaches

2) As indicated in **Table D-1**, focal muscle contraction can be identified in some individuals with tension-type headaches or cervicogenic pain.

Medication Review

3) Medication Review is required for people with headaches that have been present for more than two weeks and for individuals with frequent or daily headaches. Chronic use (particularly daily) of non-steroidal anti-inflammatory drugs (NSAIDs) or acetaminophen (alone or combined with caffeine) particularly daily, may lead to rebound headaches that are similar to tension-type headaches in character. Headaches associated with chronic NSAID/acetaminophen usage should be addressed to a headache specialist. Excessive use or rapid withdrawal of caffeine or tobacco can also trigger headaches. Particular caution is required for individuals who have frequent headaches and who state that headaches respond only to opioid medications. Such individuals should be directed to a pain clinic or headache specialist.

Sleep

4) The lack of sleep can cause or exacerbate headaches and/or light sensitivity as well as problems with many cognitive/emotional functions. Ascertain current sleep/wake cycles and provide counseling regarding appropriate sleep hygiene (limiting use of stimulants, encouraging exercise, reducing pre-sleep stimuli from lights/noise, reducing pre-sleep fluid intake, discouraging naps). Concussion is also associated with impaired sleep; i.e., disturbed abnormal breathing patterns, or disruptions in progression of sleep cycles.

Treatment

See table Appendix E for suggested list of selected medications used in treatment of headache

5) Pharmacotherapy and non-pharmacologic treatments to reduce the frequency of headaches and to treat acute headaches are based upon the character of the headaches. Patients who have mixed migraine/tension-like headaches may need treatment for both headache types. Based upon currently available information, most individuals with concussion/mTBI will have improvement in their headaches during the first 3 months of treatment. Consider referring patients who do not respond to treatments to headache specialists or pain treatment programs. It is important to maintain a positive outlook and to encourage active patient ownership and involvement in the care plan. It is also important to recognize co-morbid conditions, especially sleep disorders, anxiety disorders (PTSD) and depression. Treatment of these conditions may also improve headache.

Episodic Tension-Type Headaches

6) Episodic tension-type headaches usually respond to non-steroidal anti-inflammatory medications (NSAID) that can be obtained over-the-counter. Unfortunately, tension-type headaches associated with concussion may be resistant to medication alone. Patients may achieve better pain relief if medication treatment is coupled with other treatment modalities such as relaxation training and biofeedback. Patients should be encouraged to engage in physical therapy to exercise neck muscles and maintain appropriate range of motion. Increased physical activity may help to reduce the frequency and intensity of tension headaches. These non-pharmacologic modalities may help patients control or moderate their headaches enabling them to gain control of their pain. NSAID medications including aspirin, ibuprofen or choline-magnesium-trisalisylate and acetaminophen are the first-line medications for treating tension headaches. The choice of an NSAID or acetaminophen depends upon

individual response and severity of side effects. Aspirin is more likely to produce gastrointestinal distress and upper gastrointestinal bleeding than other NSAID medications. Acetaminophen is often the best tolerated in terms of lower likelihood to produce gastrointestinal distress. When used appropriately, side effects with acetaminophen are rare. The most serious side effect is liver damage due to large doses, chronic use or concomitant use with alcohol or other drugs that also damage the liver. Acetaminophen should be avoided in individuals with hepatitis. Choline-magnesiumtrisalisylate occasionally provides a good balance of efficacy and reduced likelihood of gastrointestinal distress. Ibuprofen can also be used to treat episodic tension headaches. If patients exhibit gastrointestinal side effects, therapy with proton-pump inhibitors and histamine blockers may be considered. Pain treatment is more likely to be successful if the medication is taken at the onset of a headache rather than waiting for the headache pain to escalate.

7) *Combination medications* can be effective in treating episodic tension headaches, but persistent usage can lead to rebound headaches. Aspirin, acetaminophen, or both are often combined with caffeine or a sedative drug in a single medication. Combination drugs may be more effective than NSAIDs or acetaminophen alone. Analgesic-sedative combinations can be obtained only by prescription because they may produce dependency, or trigger addiction in vulnerable individuals. This may lead to chronic daily headache. Combinations of acetaminophen or aspirin and an opioid should be used with great caution. These drugs should not be used more than two days a week due to concern for side effects and the potential for dependency.
8) Patients who experience more than three tension headaches per week may benefit from prophylactic therapy designed to prevent tension headaches. Poorly controlled tension headaches may indicate that attention should be directed to physical or psychological factors that may be triggering the headaches.

Migraine Headaches

9) Medical treatment of migraine headaches includes strategies for acute interventions and headache prevention. Many patients with migraine can be effectively treated with various acute headache medications and nonpharmacologic strategies. See Appendix E for list of pharmacologic treatments that can be used to treat and prevent migraine headaches. Patients need to be aware of factors that can trigger migraines and avoid those that trigger their headaches. Headache risk factors and triggers include: sleep disruption, delaying meals, stress, and, for some people, specific foods, beverages or odors can trigger migraine attacks. Nonpharmacologic treatments are often adjunctive to acute treatment although at times and especially early in the evolution of a migraine they may be effective and may eliminate the need for pharmacologic interventions. Nonpharmacologic treatments commonly employed are relaxation, biofeedback, visualization, extracranial pressure, and cold compresses. Regular exercise, maintaining regular sleep and meal schedules are an important part of the overall treatment regimen but are more effective as preventives than as treatments.
10) Interventions to reduce headache frequency should be considered when migraine headaches occur more than once a week or any of the following criteria exist:
    a) Headache attacks that are disabling despite aggressive acute interventions
    b) Patient's desire to reduce frequency of acute attacks

c) Headaches compromise work attendance, societal integration or daily life

11) Effective acute treatment requires that patients recognize their specific warning signs (aura) of an impending headache. A migraine headache often begins with mild to moderate pain that may be similar to the pain of a tension-type headache. As the migraine progresses, the headache includes the typical migraine features such as throbbing pain, nausea and phono- or photophobia. Acute treatment is more likely to succeed if medication is taken as soon as the patient recognizes the warning signs.

12) It is important that acute migraine treatment be used prudently to avoid inducing headaches due to medication overuse or rebound. Headaches associated with medication overuse are typically tension-like in character. Treatment of medication overuse headaches requires stopping daily use of acute headache medication treatment, which will lead to withdrawal symptoms that include rebound headaches. Patients can fall into a pattern of continued medication overuse to avoid rebound headaches. When patients are caught in a pattern of medication-overuse, they are usually refractory to preventive medications. In most cases, headaches improve after an analgesic washout period. It is important to educate patients that acute migraine medication treatment be limited to 3 treatments a week or less on a regular basis. A headache diary including frequency and medication history use may be useful in detecting medication overuse.

13) If acute treatment of a migraine is not effective, rescue treatment may be needed to break the migraine cycle (see **Table D-2**). If rescue therapy is required more than once a month, then the patient should receive prophylactic treatment as well as acute treatment.

Table D-2. Rescue interventions for migraine

Intervention	Comment
Medications	Due to nausea medications should be administered via injection or suppository
NSAID - Ketorolac	Gastric protection against ulceration may be considered.
Triptans or Ergotamines	These agents are available in parenteral formulations, nasal sprays and oral tablets. Given early, may abort migraine attack, may be ineffective for an advanced migraine attack.
Tramadol	The side effect of sedation can be useful as migraine attacks can abate with sleep.
Divalproex sodium	Intravenous administration of 500mg can break a migraine
Butorphanol (Stadol)	This is available in a nasal inhalation formulation; given early may be able to abort a migraine attack
Opioids	Morphine sulfate 2-4mg or comparable dose of another parenteral opioid can be useful in breaking a migraine attack. Regular usage can lead to habituation. This class of medications is usually avoided in mTBI patients.
Oxygen Inhalation	This treatment can be given in conjunction with other interventions. Oxygen is typically provided as 2-4 liters per minute via nasal prongs or mask.
Prochlorperazine	Rectal suppositories 25 mg twice daily may cause sedation
Promethazine	Rectal suppositories 12.5-25 mg every 4-6 hours as needed may cause sedation

References

Boline PD, Kassak K, Bronfort G, Nelson C, Anderson AV. Spinal manipulation vs.Amitriptyline for the treatment of chronic tension-type headaches: A randomized clinical trial. *J Manipulative Physiol Ther.* 1995;18:148-54.

Bove G, Nilsson N. Spinal manipulation in the treatment of episodic tension-type headache: A randomized controlled trial. *JAMA.* 1998;280:1576-79.

Daly CM, Doyle ME, Raskind M, Raskind E, Daniels C. Clinical case series: The use of prazosin for combat-related recurrent nightmares among operation iraqi freedom combat veterans. *Mil Med.* 2005;170:513-5

Garcia-Monco JC, Foncea N, Bilbao A, Ruiz de Velasco I, Gomez-Beldarrain M. Impact of preventive therapy with nadolol and topiramate on the quality of life of migraine patients. *Cephalgia.* 2007;27:920-8

Headache Classification Subcommittee of the International Headache Society. *The International Classification of Headache Disorders,* 2nd edition. *Cephalgia. 2004*;24 (Suppl 1):9-160.

Huffman JC, Stern TA. Neuropsychiatric consequences of cardiovascular medications. *Dialogues Clin Neurosci.* 2007;9:29-45

Kaniecki R, Lucas S. Treatment of primary headache: Preventive treatment of migraine. In: Foundation NH, ed. *Standards of care for headache diagnosis and treatment.* Chicago: National Headache Foundation, 2004:40-52

Landy S, Smith T. Treatment of primary headache: Acute migraine treatment. *Standards of care for headache diagnosis and treatment.* Chicago: National Headache Foundation, 2004:27-39.

Lew HL, Lin P-H, Fuh J-L, Wang S-J, Clark DC, Walker WC. Characteristics and Treatment of Headache After Traumatic Brain Injury: A Focused Review. *Am J Phys Med Rehabil.* 2006;85:619-27

Linder SL. Post-traumatic Headache. *Curr Pain Headache Rep.* 2007;11:396-400.

Mathew N, Ward T. Treatment of primary headache: Chronic daily headache. *Standards of care for headache diagnosis and treatment.* Chicago: National Headache Foundation, 2004:73-80.

Ramadan NM. Current trends in migraine prophylaxis. *Headache.* 2007;47 Suppl 1:S52-7

Raskind MA, Peskind ER, Hoff DJ, Hart KL, Holmes HA, Warren D, Shofer J, O'Connell J, Taylor F, Gross C, Rohde K, McFall ME. A parallel group placebo controlled study of prazosin for trauma nightmares and sleep disturbance in combat veterans with post-traumatic stress disorder. *Biol Psychiatry.* 2007;61:928-34

Ruff RL, Ruff SS, Wang X-F: Headaches Among Veterans of Operations Iraqi Freedom and Enduring Freedom with Mild Traumatic Brain Injury Associated with Exposures to Explosions. *J Rehab Res & Dev* accepted for publication, 2008.

Ruoff G, Urban G. Treatment of primary headache: Episodic tension-type headache. *Standards of care for headache diagnosis and treatment.* Chicago: National Headache Foundation, 2004:53-8.

Stoudemire A, Brown JT, Harris RT, Blessing-Feussner C, Roberts JH, Nichols JC, Houpt JL. Propranolol and depression: A reevaluation based on a pilot clinical trial. *Psychiatr Med.* 1984;2:211-8.

Taber KH, Warden DL, Hurley RA. Blast-Related Traumatic Brain Injury: What Is Known? *J Neuropsychiatry Clin Neurosci.* 2006;18:141-45

Walker WC, Seel RT, Curtiss G, Warden DL. Headache after moderate and severe traumatic brain injury: a longitudinal analysis. *Arch Phys Med Rehabil.* 2005;86:1793-800

Warden DL. Military TBI during the Iraq and Afghanistan wars. *J Head Trauma Rehabil.* 2006;21:398-402

D-2. Dizziness and Disequilibrium

Background: Dizziness and disequilibrium are common symptoms/signs of many diagnoses, concussion/mTBI being one of them. Dizziness, impaired balance and altered coordination have been reported in as many as 30% of people after mTBI (Cicerone, 1995). Dizziness and disequilibrium disorders that may result from concussion/mTBI can be organized into the following disorders: inner ear disorders (peripheral vestibular disorders), central nervous system disorders, psychological disorders and musculoskeletal disorders.

Recommendations:

ASSESSMENT

Physical Examination

1) Observation and patient interview are key elements to the exam and often guide the clinician in determining the plan of care. Evaluation should include a thorough neurologic examination and the following systems review: vision (acuity, tracking, saccades, nystagmus), auditory (hearing screen, otoscopic exam), sensory (sharp, light touch, proprioception, vibration), motor (power, coordination) and vestibular (dynamic acuity, positional testing). Evaluation of functional activities should include sitting and standing (Romberg with eyes open/closed, single leg stance) balance, transfers (supine↔sit, sit↔stand) and gait (walking, tandem walking, turning).

Table D-3. Criteria for categorization and referral for dizziness and disequilibrium after mTBI (Shumway-Cook, 2007; Shepard et al, 2007)

	Possible Diagnosis	Symptoms	Duration/Provocation	Referral
	Inner Ear Disorders (Peripheral Vestibular Disorders)			
1	Benign positional vertigo	Vertigo Lightheadedness Nausea	• Spells that last for seconds and are associated with changes in head position • Nystagmus usually observed when symptomatic	• Canalithic repositioning maneuver • Vestibular Rehabilitation
2	Labyrinthine Concussion	Vertigo with movement Disequilibrium Oscillopsia with head movements Nausea & vomiting (acute)	• History of event, symptoms improved since event but remain problematic • Mostly related to fast head movements/turns	• ENT • Physical Therapy

	Possible Diagnosis	Symptoms	Duration/Provocation	Referral
3	Post-traumatic endolymphatic hydrops	Vertigo Disequilibrium Aural fullness Tinnitus	• Spontaneous, episodic spells that can last for hours	• ENT
4	Perilymphatic fistula	Loud tinnitus Hearing loss Vertigo	• Onset related to an event • Increase in abdominal pressure can elicit symptoms	• ENT
5	Bilateral labyrinthine dysfunction	Disequilibrium Vertigo & oscillopsia if lesions asymmetrical	• Related to one or more events, induced by head movements, difficulty with postural control in the dark or on uneven surfaces	• ENT • Physical Therapy
Central Disorder				
6	Frontal lobe contusion	Decreased attention Impulsivity Imbalance Apraxia	• Postural issues related to increased attentional demands, both internal (multi-tasking) and external (environmental)	• Physiatry • Physical Therapy
7	Migraine-induced vestibulopathy	Motion sensitivity Disequilibrium Headache	• Movement induced spells of vertigo that usually last for minutes to one hour, usually close temporal relationship with headache	• See Section D-1: Headache • Physical Therapy
8	Visual dysfunction	Dizziness Disequilibrium Blurred vision Diplopia Impaired visual-spatial orientation Eye-hand incoordination Excessive peripheral vision stimulation	• Difficulties with balance on uneven, conforming terrain • Dizziness with increased environmental stimulation • Squinting/closing one eye during activities • Difficulty standing in midline or noted head tilt	• Ophthalmology • Vision Rehabilitation
Psychological Disorder				
9	Depression, anxiety, somatization	• Lightheadedness • Floating • Rocking • Vague/bizarre accounts	• May be related to event but could report chronic history, symptoms can be induced by eye movments with head still	• Psychiatry • Psychology • Physical Therapy
Musculoskeletal Disorder				
10	Flexion-extension, cervical injury (cervicogenic)	• Vertigo • Disequilibrium • Lightheadedness • Neck pain	• Onset with event • Symptoms coincide with movement of cervical spine	• Physiatry • Physical Therapy
Uncommon Central Disorders				
11	Brain stem or cerebellar dysfunction	• Vertigo • Disequilibrium • Nausea & Vomiting • Head/trunk tilt • Lateropulsion • Ataxia • Sensory disturbance • Oscillopsia • Vision deficits • Incoordination	• Onset with event • Can be exacerbated by movement	• Neurology • Physical Therapy • Ophthalmology • Vision Rehabilitation

(Continued)

	Possible Diagnosis	Symptoms	Duration/Provocation	Referral
12	Vertebral-basilar insufficiency related to occipitoatlantal instability	• Nausea & vomiting • Vertigo • Visual hallucinations/ loss • Visual field deficit • Numbness/weakness • Ataxia • Drop attacks	• Related to an event • Usually symptoms induced by cervical extension and rotation	• Neurology • Neurosurgery
		• Diplopia • Headaches		
13	Temporal bone fracture	• Conductive hearing loss • Vertigo • Disequilibrium • Nausea & vomiting • Oscillopsia	• Onset with event • Will follow the course of labyrinthine concussion	• ENT • Physical Therapy

Medication Review

2) A detailed medication history is warranted. Numerous medications include dizziness as a potential side effect. The following classes of medication can cause or aggravate dizziness: stimulants, benzodiazepines, tricyclics, monoamine oxidase inhibitors, tetracyclics, neuroleptics, anticonvulsants, selective serotonin agonists, beta blockers and cholinesterase inhibitors. The temporal relationship to the onset of dizziness and the initiation/dosing of these medications should be investigated.

Treatment:

Pharmacologic Treatment

3) Initiating vestibular suppressants for dizziness may delay central compensation or promote counterproductive compensation (Hain & Yacovino, 2005; Pyykko I, 1988). Vestibular suppressants might be helpful during the acute period of several vestibular disorders but have not been shown to be effective in chronic dizziness after concussion (Zee, 1985). Medications should only be considered if symptoms are severe enough to significantly limit functional activities. Trials should be limited to 2 weeks. With concussion/mTBI be particularly careful regarding dosing and titration due to the effects on arousal and memory as well as potential addictive qualities of these medications (Arciniegas, 2005).

   First line medication choice would be meclizine, followed by scopolamine and dimenhydrinate depending upon symptom presentation. Pharmacotherapy with clonazepam, diazepam or lorazepam should be carefully considered due to their sedating and addictive qualities. (See Table D-6)

Non-Pharmacologic Treatment

4) Non-pharmacologic interventions for post-traumatic dizziness may be useful as an alternative to pharmacotherapies (de Kruijk et al., 2002), although the effectiveness of such interventions is not fully established with concussion/mTBI. Efficacy of vestibular and balance rehabilitation has been found in different populations with vestibular disorders (Herdman et al., 1995; Shepard & Telian, 1995; Yardley et al., 1998). Patients with vestibular disorders who received customized programs showed greater improvement than those who received generic exercises (Shepard & Telian,

1995). Studies utilizing vestibular exercises have shown up to 85% success rate in reducing symptoms and improving function in the population with peripheral vestibular disorders (Krebs et al, 2003; Shepard & Telian, 1995). With concussion/mTBI, recovery of vestibular lesions is often limited or protracted due to the coexistence of central or psychological disorders (Gottshall et al., 2007).

5) Knowledge of the canalith repositioning procedures (Fife, 2008) for the treatment of benign positional vertigo would be beneficial for primary care physicians. The types of exercise to treat dizziness and disequilibrium are beyond the scope of this guideline. Central and psychological disorders need a coordinated team effort to address the underlying impairments to maximize outcome of vestibular rehabilitation.

Evidence Statement

- Concussion/mTBI in the acute stage may cause dizziness (Ernst, 2005; Hoffer, 2004; Staab, 2007) [Level of Evidence = B]
- Subjective reports of dizziness correlate with objective testing only during the first week post-injury of concussion/mTBI (Gottshall, 2007). [Level of Evidence = B]
- Concussion/mTBI may cause coordination deficits of the lower extremities (imbalance) and/or upper extremities (dysmetria) (Catena, 2007, Heitger, 2006; Parker, 2006) [Level of Evidence = B]
- Cognitive distractions or performance of dual tasks are sensitive provocative tests for detection of imbalance and coordination deficits in the acute stage of Concussion/mTBI (Catena, 2006; Parker, 2006) [Level of Evidence = B]
- Adjusted for age, gender, educational and employment status, concussion/mTBI patients who had dizziness and/or headache were almost three fold more likely to develop persistent symptoms at one month (Savola & Hillborn, 2003). [Level of Evidence = C]
- Some evidence suggests that vestibular rehabilitation may improve post-traumatic dizziness symptoms (Hoffer, 2004) [Level of Evidence = C]

References

Arciniegas DB, Anderson CA, Topkoff J, McAllister TW. Mild traumatic brain injury: A neuropsychiatric approach to diagnosis, evaluation, and treatment. *Neuropsychiatric* Disease And Treatment 2005;1:311-327

Catena R. van Donkelaar P. Chou L. Altered balance control following concussion is better detected with an attention test during gait. *Gait & Posture* 2006 (25) 406-411.

Cicerone KD, Kalmar K. Persistent post concussive syndrome: the structure of subjective complaints after mild traumatic brain injury. *J Head Trauma Rehabil* 1995;10(3):1-17.

de Kruijk JR, Leffers P, Meerhoff S, Rutten J, Twijnstra A. Effectiveness of bed rest after mild traumatic brain injury: a randomised trial of no versus six days of bed rest. *J Neurol Neurosurg Psychiatry 2002*;73:167-172

Ernst A, Basta D, Seidl RO, et al. Management of posttraumatic vertigo. *Otolaryngol Head Neck Surg* 2005;132:554-558

Fife TD et al. Practice Parameters: Therapies for benign paroxysmal positional vertigo. *Neurology* 2008; 70:2067-74.

Gottshall, KR et al. To investigate the influence of acute vestibular impairment following mild traumatic brain injury on subsequent ability to remain on active duty 12 months later. *Military Medicine.* 2007;172(8): 852-7.

Hain TC, Yacovino D. Pharmacologic treatment of persons with dizziness. *Neurol Clin* 2005;23:831- 853.

Heitger MH, Jones RD, Dalrymple-Alford JC, et al. Motor deficits and recovery during the first year following mild closed head injury. *Brain Inj* 2006;20:807-824

Herdman SJ et al. Vestibular adaptation exercises and recovery: acute stage after acoustic neuroma resection. *Otolaryngol Head Neck Surg* 1995;113:77-87.

Hoffer ME, Gottshall KR, Moore R, Balough BJ, Wester D. Characterizing and treating dizziness after mild head trauma. *Otology & Neurotology* 2004;25:135-138

Krebs DE et al. Vestibular rehabilitation: useful but not universally so. *Otolaryngol Head Neck Surg* 2003;128:240-50.

Parker TM, Osternig LR, Van Donkelaar P, Chou LS. Gait stability following concussion. *Medicine and Science in Sports and Exercise* 2006;38:1032-1040

Pyykko I, et al. Pharmacological treatment of vertigo. *Acta Otolaryngol Suppl* 1988;455:77-81.

Shepard NT, Clendaniel RA, Ruckenstein M. Balance and dizziness. In: Zasler ND, Katz DI, Zafonte RD, eds. *Brain Injury Medicine.* New York: Demos; 2007.

Shephard NT, Telian SA. Programmatic vestibular rehabilitation. *Otolaryngol Head Neck Surg* 1995;112:173-82.

Staab JP, Ruckenstein MJ. Expanding the differential diagnosis of chronic dizziness. *Arch Otolaryngol Head Neck Surg* 2007;133:170-176

Shumway-Cook A: Assessment and management of the patient with traumatic brain injury and vestibular dysfunction. In: Herdman SJ, ed. *Vestibular Rehabilitation*, 3rd. Philadelphia: FA Davis; 2007.

Yardley L et al. A randomized controlled trial of exercise therapy for dizziness and vertigo in primary care. *Br J Gen Pract* 1998;48:1136-40.

Zee DS. Perspectives on the pharmacotherapy of vertigo. *Arch Otolaryngol* 1985;111(9):609-12.

D-3. Fatigue

Background: Fatigue is the third most common symptom reported in concussion/mTBI. It can be due to a primary effect related to central nervous system dysfunction or a secondary effect such as common co-existing disorders in concussion/mTBI such as depression or sleep disturbances. Medications, substance use and lifestyle may also contribute to fatigue.

Recommendations:

Assessment

1) A detailed history looking at pre/post-injury level of physical activity, cognitive function and mental health is important to determine the effects of fatigue in relation to the injury. The ability to maintain a job is often a good measure of the impact of

this symptom. Several outcome measures exist for fatigue and many have been studied in other diagnostic populations. Common measures in TBI include the Multidimensional Assessment of Fatigue (MAF), Fatigue Impact Scale (FIS) or Fatigue Assessment Instrument (FAI.) For concussion/mTBI there is no specific scale recommended. Laboratory tests may include blood count, metabolic panel, vitamin B12 and folate levels, thyroid function test and Erythrocyte Sedimentation Rate (ESR).

Medication Review

2) Due to the large number of centrally acting medications, a medication review is necessary. If a medication appears contributory, performance of an Applied Behavioral Analysis (ABA) trial is indicated to determine the association. Review of illicit drugs, alcohol, tobacco and caffeine/other stimulants should be performed.

Table D-4. Criteria for Characterizing Fatigue

Effect	Assessment	Treatment
Metabolic (uncommon in concussion/mTBI)	Positive lab findings	Further medical evaluation
Physical	Usually subjective, state of weariness related to physical exertion resulting in diminished capacity for work or decreased response to stimuli	Individualized fitness program
Cognitive	Usually subjective, state of weariness related to increased mental effort resulting in diminished capacity for work or decreased response to stimuli	Cognitive rehabilitation (Educational Programming, Cognitive Behavioral Therapy)
Sleep Disturbance	Self-reported, Positive sleep studies	See section D-4 Sleep Disorder
Depression	Depression screen	See Algorithm C: Persistent Emotional and cognitive Symptom management

Treatment

Pharmacologic Treatment

3) All medical and psychological disorders underlying fatigue should be treated. Modifiable factors should be addressed and typical conservative measures taken prior to initiating pharmacotherapy for fatigue. Several stimulants have had success in other disease states associated with fatigue. Although widely used in TBI, there is limited evidence in use of these medications for treatment of fatigue in concussion/mTBI.

   If symptoms have persisted for more than 4 weeks post-injury and the fatigue level has not improved with the management of sleep, pain, depression, or lifestyle, then a neurostimulant may be tried. (See Appendix E)

   Medication trials should persist for at least 3 months. Use of neurostimulant medications is contraindicated if there is a history of substance abuse.

Non-Pharmacologic Treatment

4) Education is important in the treatment of fatigue. Educational efforts should be in the areas of factors contributing to fatigue, importance of well balanced meals, promotion of sleep hygiene and regular exercise. Exercise routines should be

individualized to maximize benefit and promote proper ratio of activity/rest. Scheduling of exercise may need to be addressed depending upon when the patient is at his or her best. Cognitive-behavioral and physical therapy can be tried to decrease fatigue level and improve functional performance in patients with concussion/mTBI.

Evidence Statements

- Several studies have demonstrated the association between concussion/mTBI and fatigue (Borgaro et al., 2005; Stulemeijer et al., 2006; 2006b).
- There is some evidence to supports that multiple concussion/mTBI-related and -non related factors contribute to fatigue (Stulemeijer 2006; Stulemeijer 2006b; Ziino et al, 2005). That association is not related to the severity of TBI (Borgaroet al., 2005).
- In a controlled descriptive study, patients with concussion reported greater fatigue than those in the control group despite similar levels of mood disorders (Lachapelle, 1998; Zinio et al, 2005).
- Persistent post-concussion fatigue is related to early fatigue symptoms but can also develop over time (Norrie et al, 2007).
- There is no research evidence to support a specific treatment regimen for fatigue, however management of associated factors (e.g., mood, sleep, pain, medication effect) has been advocated (Borgaro et al, 2005; Stulemeijer et al., 2006a, 2007; Ziino et al, 2005).
- There is research evidence to support improvement of fatigue symptoms after mTBI during the first 6 months (Borg et al, 2004; Stulemeijer et al., 2006b).
- Several pharmacologic agents have been trialed in TBI with variable success. A recent study in the population with TBI found that there was no consistent or persistent clinical significance with use of modafinil over placebo (Jha, 2008.)

References

Borg J, Holm L, Peloso P M, et al; Non-Surgical Intervention and Cost for Mild Traumatic brain Injury: Results of the WHO Collaborating Centre Task Force on Mild Traumatic Brain Injury; *J. Rehabil Med;* Suppl. 43, 76-83; 2004

Borgaro, S.R., et al.,(2005). Subjective Reports of Fatigue During Early Recovery From Traumatic Brain Injury. *Journal of Head Trauma Rehabilitation,* 20(5): p. 416-425.

Jha A et al. A randomized trial of Modafinil for the treatment of fatigue and excessive daytime sleepiness in individuals with chronic traumatic brain injury. *J Head Trauma Rehabil* 2008;23(1):52-63.

Lachapelle DL, Finlayson MAJ. An evaluation of subjective and objective measures of fatigue in patients with brain injury and healthy controls. *Brain Injury* 1998;12:649-659

Norrie J, Heitger M, Leathem J, Anderson T, Jones R. Fatigue and post-concussion syndrome following mild traumatic brain injury: A preliminary report from a New Zealand sample. *Australian Journal of Psychology* 2006;58:172-173

Norrie JM, Heitger MH, Leathem JM, Anderson TJ, Jones RD. Mild traumatic brain injury and fatigue: Preliminary findings from a longitudinal prospective study. *Clinical Neuropsychologist* 2007;21:401-401

Stulemeijer M, van der Werf S, Bleijenberg G, Biert J, Brauer J, Vos PE. Recovery from mild traumatic brain injury: a focus on fatigue. *J Neurol* 2006;253:1041-7.

Stulemeijer M, Vos PE, Bleijenberg G, van der Werf SP. Cognitive complaints after mild traumatic brain injury: Things are not always what they seem. *Journal of Psychosomatic Research* 2007;63:637-45.

Stulemeijer M, van der Werf SP, Jacobs B, et al. Impact of additional extracranial injuries on outcome after mild traumatic brain injury. *J Neurotrauma* 2006b;23:1561-9.

Ziino C, Ponsford J. Measurement and prediction of subjective fatigue following traumatic brain injury. *J Int Neuropsychol Soc* 2005;11:416-425

D-4. Sleep Dysfunction

Background: Sleep disturbance often occurs acutely after concussion. Persistent difficulty falling asleep or staying asleep despite the opportunity (insomnia) is a common symptom of post trauma. Concussion/mTBI might contribute to the emergence of circadian rhythm sleep disorders. Two types of these disorders have been observed: delayed sleep phase syndrome and irregular sleep–wake pattern. Sleep apnea, depression, pain, and other conditions may contribute to the overall poor quality of sleep. (See Table D-5 Management of Sleep Dysfunction)

Recommendations:

1) Pharmacological approaches to sleep regulation may prove beneficial. (See Appendix E)
2) Cognitive behavioral sleep interventions have also been shown to be effective in normalizing sleep, these might include sleep restriction, sleep hygiene education, relaxation training and others. The goals of sleep management should be to establish a regular, unbroken, night-time sleep pattern and to improve perceptions of the quality of sleep.
3) If a patient with concussion/mTBI has a concurrent *primary* sleep disorder (e.g., sleep apnea, restless leg syndrome, or narcolepsy) a specific appropriate intervention may be required.
4) The aim of sleep management is to establish a regular, normalized sleep-wake pattern. Patients should be encouraged to:

- Avoid alcohol
- Restrict the night-time sleep period to about eight hours
- Avoid going to bed too early in the evening
- Avoid stimulants, caffeinated beverages, power drinks, and nicotine during the evening period
- Arise from bed at a regular time in the morning (e.g., by 8 a.m.)
- Wake at a regular time in the morning (e.g., 7 a.m.)
- Reduce (to less than 30 minutes) or abolish daytime naps
- Engage in daytime physical and mental activities (within the limits of the individual's functional capacity)
- Avoid stimulating activities before bedtime (e.g., exercise, video games, T.V.)

Table D-5. Management of Sleep Dysfunction

Acute Phase	Chronic Phase (>3 months).
○ Provide education about concussion with regard to changes in sleep quality and duration sometimes associated with concussion.	○ Review current medications and other current health conditions for factors which might contribute to chronic sleep disturbances, including chronic pain. Provide information about the potential effects of medications, caffeine, tobacco, and alcohol on sleep.
○ Provide information on good sleep habits with specific suggestions to improve the quality and duration of sleep, e.g., regularly scheduled bedtime.	○ Evaluate for potential co-morbid psychiatric conditions, including depression and anxiety and, if present, consider using standard medications which may improve sleep.
○ Provide information about the potential effects of medications, caffeine, tobacco, and alcohol on sleep.	○ If patient has a chronic pain disorder, appropriate pain management may assist with improving sleep duration and quality.
○ Sleep medications may be helpful in the short-term (non-benzodiapenes).	○ Consider sleep study to provide objective evidence of sleep disturbance and to rule out coexisting sleep apnea or other sleep disorders.
	○ Training in behavioral techniques, such as relaxation training or meditation to improve the quality of sleep.
	○ Consider a course of Cognitive Behavioral Therapy (CBT) focused on sleep with additional behavioral interventions to include Sleep Restriction, Stimulus Control and Relapse Prevention Techniques.

For additional recommendations –See VHA Pharmacy Benefit Management (PBM) guideline for Insomnia:

http://www.pbm.va.gov/guidelines/Treatment%20of%20Acute-Chronic %20Insomnia-Guidance%20for%20Tx%20of%20Insomnia%20in%20 Primary%20Care%20Setting -Recommendation%20for%20Use%20Zolpidem%20IR.doc

Patient Resources for Basic Hygiene Education

http://www.womenshealth.gov/faq/insomnia.htm#5

http://www.aasmnet.org/FactSheet.aspx

http://www.sleepfoundation.org/

Example of a sleep diary:

http://www.nhlbi.nih.gov/health/prof/sleep/insom_pc.pdf

Professional Education:

http://www.sleepfoundation.org/

http://www.ahrq.gov/clinic/epcsums/insomnsum.htm

D-5. Persistent Pain

(See also D-1 for a complete discussion of headache pain)

Background: Pain other than headache pain is common in patients with concussion/mTBI. Musculoskeletal pain is a common comorbid condition in concussion. Evaluating pain and treating it symptomatically is important as pain is associated with poor outcomes in TBI. Pain can be caused by any of a number of co-morbid conditions as well as musculoskeletal injuries or secondary damage to soft tissue.

Assessing patients for pain and its underlying causes is an essential component of the clinical work-up. It is important to attribute symptoms correctly and to identify and treat any comorbid conditions. If medication is being considered, it is essential that the underlying cause has been established prior to prescribing.

Recommendations:

1) Pain management must be a priority and all patients presenting with concussion should be assessed for pain on a regular basis.
2) Choice of treatment modalities for patients with concussion should be based upon risk benefit.
3) Pain management for patients with concussion should be based on a patient-centered model of care.
4) A pain management plan must consider the causation, psychosocial factors and general physical condition of the patient with concussion.
5) Effective drugs for pain relief for the patient with concussion include nonsteroidal anti-inflammatory drugs (NSAIDs), or muscle relaxants.
6) Physical therapy may be beneficial in conjunction with medications for the patient with concussion.

References

Alfano D. P., Asmundson G. J. G., Larsen D. K., Allerdings M. D.Mild traumatic brain injury and chronic pain: preliminary findings *Archives of Clinical Neuropsychology,* Volume 15, Issue 8, , November 2000, Pages 831-832

Borczuk, P.: Mild head trauma. Emergency Medicine Clinics of North America, 15: 563-579, 1997. Kraus, JF, Nourjah, P.: The epidemiology of mild uncomplicated brain injury. *J Trauma.* 28:1,637-1643, 1988

Borg J, Holm L, Cassidy J, et al. Diagnostic procedures in mild traumatic brain injury: results of the WHO Collaborating Centre Task Force on Mild Traumatic Brain Injury. *J Rehabil Med* 2004; (43 Suppl):61–75.

Nampiaparampil DE. Prevalence of chronic pain after traumatic brain injury: a systematic review. *JAMA.* 2008 Aug 13;300(6):711-9.

NIH Consensus Development Panel on Rehabilitation of Persons with Traumatic Brain Injury. Rehabilitation of persons with traumatic brain injury. *JAMA* 1999 282(10):974–8

D-6. Management of Other Symptoms

The following recommendations for treatment of other physical symptoms, less common in patients presenting with concussion/mTBI symptoms, were formulated based on consensus of clinical experts.

Vision Difficulties

Background: Vision difficulties, including sensitivity to light, diplopia, blurring and other difficulties seeing, occur acutely in up to half of all individuals who sustain a concussion. Symptoms are either blurring of vision ("double vision") that worsens over the course of the day or difficulty with visual stimulation with resultant pain (headache, eye ache) or sensitivity. The vast majority resolve within a month. Aggressive, focal treatments aimed at symptom management (reassurance, pain management, controlling environmental light, sunglasses, intermittent patching for double vision) in the first 4-6 weeks are usually effective. True abnormalities in visual acuity, visual fields or structural damage the eye are extremely rare with mTBI. Other causes of problems are also extremely rare and often not related directly to the concussion injury. Pre-injury visual deficits are common and need to be ruled out.

Recommendations:

1) Perform an ophthalmologic examination to include extraocular movements, pupils and visual fields by confrontation.
2) Refer to optometry and/or ophthalmology as indicated.
3) Allow initial use (until in therapy) of sunglasses and then give formal weaning program (decrease by 15 minutes every 2 hours).
4) Consider non-organic vision loss in patients who present with prolonged sunglass use even in low light settings.

Hearing Difficulties

Background: Hearing difficulties, including altered acuity and sensitivity to noise, occur acutely in up to three-quarters of all individuals who sustain a blast related concussion. Symptoms are either of decreased auditory acuity or sensitivity to noise. The vast majority of those symptoms resolve within a month, unless there is significant or permanent injury to the ear drum. Aggressive, focal treatments aimed at symptom management (reassurance, pain management, controlling environmental noise, white noise generators) in the first 4-6 weeks are usually effective. True abnormalities in central auditory acuity or processing are extremely rare with mTBI. Other causes of problems are also extremely rare and often not related directly to the concussion injury. Pre-injury hearing deficits are common and need to be ruled out.

Recommendations:

1) Perform an otologic examination.
2) Review medications for ototoxicity.
3) Refer to audiology for hearing assessment if no other apparent cause is found.

Smell (Olfactory Deficits)

Background: Post-traumatic olfactory deficits (anosmia) are not common in individuals who sustain a concussion, occurring in less than 25%. Symptoms are typically seen with a decreased appetite, but this may be a sign of a significant injury to the frontal lobe and other central difficulties must be ruled out. The vast majority resolve within a 6 month period. Treatments have limited effect and are usually aimed at flavoring/spicing food to enhance taste. Other causes are also extremely rare and often not related directly to the concussion injury. Pre-injury causes of anosmia need to be ruled out.

Recommendations

1. Perform a nasal and oropharyngeal examination and depression screen.
2. Refer to ENT for further evaluation if needed.
3. If neurologic status is stable and no objective findings then reassurance and monitoring is appropriate. Increase spicing of foods (+/- dietary referral). Monitor weights.

Changes in Appetite

Background: Post-traumatic appetite deficits are not common in individuals who sustain a concussion, occurring in less than 5%. When a change in appetite is noted, it may be related to mood, medications, smell, or other factors and will likely resolve. Treatments have limited effect and are usually aimed at flavoring/spicing food to enhance taste or managing depression. Other causes are also extremely rare and often not related directly to the concussion injury. Pre-injury causes of appetite issues need to be ruled out.

Recommendations

1) Perform nasal and oropharyngeal examination.
2) Review neurovegetative signs with patient to assess for depressed affect or clinical depression.
3) Assess medication list for agents that can cause olfactory or gustatory abnormalities (centrally acting medications, in particular anti-epileptics, some antibiotics).
4) If neurologic status is stable and no objective findings then reassurance and monitoring is appropriate. Increase spicing of foods (+/- dietary referral). Monitor weights.

Numbness

It is extremely rare to see numbness with mTBI in the absence of peripheral nerve injury, and it usually represents somatization. If neurologic status is stable and no objective findings then reassurance and monitoring is appropriate.

Recommendation:

1. Perform a sensory examination.

Nausea

Background: Post-traumatic nausea occurs occasionally acutely after concussion, most often in combination with dizziness, as a secondary effect of medications (pain), or due to an exacerbation of underlying GERD/GI dysfunction. Assessment initially is limited and focus should be on rapid management of dizziness and return to activity.

Recommendations

1) Define triggers and patterns of nausea.
2) Assess medication list for agents that may cause or worsen GI symptoms.
3) Perform oropharyngeal examination.

Appendix E: Pharmacotherapy

Pharmacotherapy in Concussion/mTBI – List of Selected First line Agents

	Potential side effects	**Contraindications/ Comments**	**Common issues in concussion/mTBI**
Stimulants (In specialty care after ruling out sleep disorder.)			
First line agents: Methylphenidate 5 mg every 8 am and 1 pm, increasing total daily dose by 5 mg every 2 weeks to a maximum of 20 mg twice daily	○ Insomnia ○ Decreased appetite ○ GI upset ○ Headaches ○ Dizziness ○ Motor tics ○ Irritability ○ Anxiousness ○ Tearfulness	Ongoing substance abuse.	Possible addiction potential Requires additional prescription regulation under federal/state law. Cannot be refilled, only one month of therapy at a time may be prescribed
Modafanil start with 100 mg every morning. Increase in 100 mg amounts, using split daily dosing up to maximum of 400 mg/day	○ Headache, asthesia		
Amantadine 100-400 mg daily	○ Nausea ○ Dizziness ○ Dry mouth		
Antidepressants			
First line agents: Citalopram 10 mg daily for 1 week, then 20 mg daily if tolerated (up to 80 mg daily if needed) Sertraline 25 mg daily increasing weekly in 25 mg increments to maximum dose of 200 mg/day	○ Nausea ○ Insomnia ○ Agitation ○ Asthesia ○ Nausea ○ Insomnia ○ Dry mouth ○ Headache	Do not initiate concomitant therapy with a benzodiazepine	May cause sexual dysfunction
Non-benzodiazepine Sleep Agents			
First line agent: Zolpidem 5 mg at night, if poor results after 3 nights of therapy increase to 10 mg nightly			
Prazosin initiate therapy with 1 mg at bedtime for three days. May increase to 2 mg at bedtime through day 7.	○ Orthostatic hypotension		For patients with nightmares and/or violent or outburst or agitation during sleep
If patients continued to have nightmares, the dosage may be increased to 4 mg at bedtime through day 14.			

	Potential side effects	Contraindications/ Comments	Common issues in concussion/mTBI
The dosage could be increased to 6 mg at bedtime through day 21 and to 10 mg at bedtime through day 28.The maximum daily dose is 10 mg at bedtime.			
NSAIDS for headache			
Ibuprofen 400-600 mg three to four times daily **Naproxen** 500 mg twice daily	○ GI upset ○ Dizziness ○ vertigo		Potential renal impairment with long term use Rebound headache may occur with continuous use
Abortive agents for migraine/migraine-like headaches			
Zolmitriptan oral 5-10 mg at onset of headache, may repeat once if headache is not resolved in 2 hours **Zolmitriptan nasal** one spray of 5 mg for the treatment of acute migraine. If the headache returns the dose may be repeated after 2 hours. The maximum daily dose should not exceed 10 mg in any 24-hour period	○ unusual taste (nasal formulation), paresthesia, hyperesthesia, dizziness, chest tightness		Serious cardiac events, including myocardial infarction, have occurred following the use of zolmitriptan and sumatriptan tablets and nasal spray.
	Potential side effects	Contraindications/ Comments	Common issues in concussion/mTBI
Sumatriptan oral 50-100 mg at onset of headache, may repeat once if headache is not resolved in 2 hours **Sumatriptan nasal** 10 mg spray in one nostril, may repeat in 2 hrs not to exceed 40 mg/day **Sumatriptan injectable** 6 mg injected subcutaneously may repeat in 1 hour. Not to exceed 12 mg/day	○ Dizziness, vertigo, tingling, hypertension, injection site reactions,		These events are extremely rare and most have been reported in patients with risk factors predictive of CAD
Prophylactic headache agents			
First line agents: **Divalproex sodium extended release** 250 mg twice daily, increase by 250 mg/day every week to a maximum of 1000 mg/day	○ Asthenia, dizziness, somnolence, tremor, nausea, diplopia	Hepatic failure resulting in fatalities has occurred in patients receiving valproic acid and its derivatives	May take up to 3 months to receive the full benefit from any of the prophylactic medications Association with teratogenecity, neural tube effects. Caution in women of childbearing potential
Topiramate 25-100 mg twice daily	○ Anorexia, sedation, ataxia, dizziness		May worsen cognitive dysfunction May cause renal stones
Metoprolol initiate with 25 mg twice daily, increase dose up to 100 mg twice daily if needed, wait 3-4 weeks between dose increases	○ Somnolence ○ Cold extremities ○ bradycardia	There are two formulations- tartrate is immediate release, dosed 2 times daily and succinate is sustained release, dosed one time daily.	Use with caution in asthmatic and diabetic patients
Vestibular Suppressants			
Meclizine 12.5-50 mg every 4-6 hours	○ Hallucinations, blurred vision	All of the agents may cause sedation and require caution when driving or operating machinery	
Scopolamine 0.5 mg patch every 3 days	○ Dry mouth ○ Topical Allergy ○ Tachyarrhythmia		
Dimenhydrinate 50 mg every 4-6 hours orally	○ Dry mouth		
Lorazepam 0.5 mg twice a day orally **Clonazepam** 0.25 -0.5 mg twice a day orally **Diazepam** 2-10 mg orally, IM, or IV	○ Drug dependence ○ Respiratory depressant		Avoid use of benzodiazapines in mTBI if at all possible

Appendix F: Education Intervention Studies

Education and Support Intervention Studies with Mild TBI Patients

First Author	Design	Treatment(s) Tested	Study Sample	Control and Tx Groups	Follow-Up Period	Tx Better Than Control?
Mittenberg et al., 1996	RCT	Handout + one-hour session	Hospitalized after mild TBI	N = 29 N = 29	6 months	Yes
Relander et al., 1972	RCT	Activity encouraged; good prognosis emphasized	Within 36 hours of hospitalization	N=96 N=82	1 year	Yes
Minderhoud et al., 1980	Retrospective comparison	Printed + verbal education + activity encouraged	Hospitalized after mild TBI	N=352 N=180	6 months	Yes
Gronwall, 1986	Not randomized	Printed education	Within 2 weeks of injury	N=54 N=34	3 months	No
Alves et al., 1993	RCT	1. Education only 2. Education + reassurance about recovery	Hospitalized after mild TBI	N=210 N=176 N=201	3, 6, 12 months	Yes*
Ferguson & Mitenberg, 1996 as reported in Miller & Mittenberg, 1998	Case Description	12-session manualized cognitive-behavioral treatment	Referrals to outpatient clinic	N=4	12 weeks	Yes
Wade et al., 1998	RCT	Printed and verbal education + continued support	7 to 10 days post-injury	N=130 N=184	6 months	Yes
Paniak et al., 2000	RCT	Single session education	Hospital emergency room	N=59 N=60	3 to 4 months	Yes**
Tiersky et al., 2005	RCT with multiple baselines	CBT+cognitive treatment for 11 weeks	Average of 5 years post-injury	N=7 (milds) N=11	1 and 3 months	Yes
Ghaffar et al., 2006	RCT	Multidiscipline treatment	Within 1 week of injury	N=94 N=97	6 months	No
Mittenberg, 2001	SR	Booklet guide	varied	N=1014	6 months	Yes
Ponford, 2002	CT	Provision of booklet	202	C= 123 N= 79	1 week and 3 months	Yes

Notes: *For reassurance treatment group only, assuming that patients not seen at follow-up are asymptomatic. **No differences in outcomes between single session and extensive outpatient therapy. RCT = randomized control trial; CBT = cognitive behavioral therapy; Tx = Treatment.

References

Alves W, Macciocchi S, Barth J. Postconcussive symptoms after uncomplicated mild head injury. *Journal of Head Trauma Rehabilitation* 1993;8(3):48-59.

Ferguson RJ, Mittenberg W. Cognitive-behavioral treatment of postconcussion syndrome: A therapist's manual. In: Van Hasselt VB, Hersen M, editors. *Sourcebook of psychological treatment manuals for adult disorders*. New York: Plenum Press, 1996:615-655.

Ghaffar O, McCullagh S, Ouchterlony D, Feinstein A. Randomized treatment trial in mild traumatic brain injury. *Journal of Psychosomatic Research* 2006;61(2):153-60.

Gronwall D. Rehabilitation programs for patients with mild head injury: Components, problems, and evaluation. *Journal of Head Trauma Rehabilitation* 1986;1:53-63.

Miller LJ, Mittenberg W. Brief cognitive behavioral interventions in mild traumatic brain injury. *Applied Neuropsychology* 1998;5(4):172-83.

Minderhoud JM, Boelens ME, Huizenga J, Saan RJ. Treatment of minor head injuries. *Clinical Neurology and Neurosurgery* 1980;82(2):127-40.

Mittenberg W, Tremont G, Zielinski RE, Fichera S, Rayls KR. Cognitive-behavioral prevention of postconcussion syndrome. *Archives of Clinical Neuropsychology* 1996;11 (2):139-45.

Mittenberg W, Canyock E, Condit O, Patton C. Treatment of post-concussion syndrome following mild head injury. *J Clin Exper Neuropsych* 2001;23(6):829-36.

Paniak C, Toller-Lobe G, Reynolds S, Melnyk A, Nagy J. A randomized trial of two treatments for mild traumatic brain injury: 1 year follow-up. *Brain Injury* 2000;14(3):219-26.

Ponsford J, Willmott C, Rothwell A, et al. Impact of early intervention on outcome following mild head injury in adults. *Journal of Neurology Neurosurgery and Psychiatry* 2002;73:330-2.

Relander M, Troupp H, Bjorkesten G. Controlled trial of treatment for cerebral concussion. *British Medical Journal* 1972;4:777-779.

Tiersky LA, Anselmi V, Johnston MV, Kurtyka J, Roosen E, Schwartz T, et al. A trial of neuropsychologic rehabilitation in mild-spectrum traumatic brain injury. *Archives of Physical Medicine and Rehabilitation* 2005;86(8):1565-74.

Wade DT, King NS, Wenden FJ, Crawford S, Caldwell FE. Routine follow up after head injury: a second randomised controlled trial. *Journal of Neurology, Neurosurgery and Psychiatry* 1998;65(2):177-83.

Appendix G: Acronym List

ACRM	American College of Rehabilitation Medicine
ADL	Activities of Daily Living
ATC	Assistive Technology for Cognition
AOC	Alteration of Consciousness/Mental State
CAM	Complementary Alternative Medicine
CDC	Centers for Disease Control and Prevention
CT	Computed Tomography
DVBIC	Defense and Veterans Brain Injury Center
DSM-IV	Diagnostic and Statistical Manual for Mental Disorders – Fourth Edition
GCS	Glasgow Coma Score
IADL	Instrumental Activities of Daily Living
ICD-10	International Classification of Diseases - 10th Revision
LOC	Level of Consciousness
MSA	Mental Status Examination
mTBI	Mild Traumatic Brain Injury
PCD	Post-Concussion Disorder

PCS	Post-Concussion Syndrome or Post Concussive Syndrome
PPCS	Persistent Post Concussive Symptoms
PTA	Post-Traumatic Amnesia
PTSD	Post-Traumatic Stress Disorder
OIF/OEF	Operations Iraqi Freedom and Enduring Freedom
SR	Strength of the Recommendation
USPSTF	United States Preventative Services Task Force
WHO	World Health Organization

Appendix H: Participant List

Jeffrey Barth Ph.D., ABPP-CN
John Edward Fowler Professor
Head, Neurocognitive Study Section
Director, Brain Injury and Sports Concussion Institute
Neurocognitive Assessment Laboratory
Dept. of Psychiatry and Neurobehavioral Sciences
University of Virginia School of Medicine
Box 800203 HS
Charlottesville, VA. 22908
Phone:434-924-2718
Email:JTB4Y@hscmail.mcc.virginia.edu

Kathleen R. Bell, MD
University of Washington
Department of Rehabilitation Medicine
1959 NE Pacific Street
Box 356490
Seattle, WA 98195-6490
krbell@u.washington.edu
Phone: 206-685-0935
Email: krbell@u.washington.edu

Amy Bowles, MD
Chief, Traumatic Brain Injury Service
Physical Medicine and Rehabilitation Department
Brooke Army Medical Center
3851 Roger Brooke Drive
Fort Sam Houston, TX 78234-6200
Phone: 210-916-8693
Email: amy.bowles@amedd.army.mil

Carla Cassidy, RN, MSN, NP
Director, Evidence Based Practice Program
Department of Veterans Affairs
810 Vermont Avenue
Washington, DC 20420
Phone: (202) 266-4502
Email: Carla.cassidy@va.gov

David Cifu, MD
Chief, Physical Medicine and Rehabilitation Department
Hunter Holmes McGuire VA Medical Center
1201 Broad Rock Boulevard
Richmond, VA 23249
Phone: 804-675-5117
Email: david.cifu@va.gov or dcifu@vcu.edu

Douglas Cooper, PhD
Clinical Neuropsychologist
Traumatic Brain injury Service
Department of Orthopedics & Rehabilitation
Brooke Army Medical Center
3851 Roger Brooke Drive
Fort Sam Houston,TX 78234-6200
Phone: 210-916-3955
Email: douglas.cooper2@amedd.army.mil

Ernest Degenhardt, RN, MSN, ANP-FNP
COL, USA
Chief, Evidence-Based Practice
Quality Management Division
US Army Medical Command
2050 Worth Road, Suite 26
Fort Sam Houston TX 78234
Phone:210-221-6527 or DSN 471-6527
Email: ernest.degenhardt@amedd.army.mil

Martha D'Erasmo, MPH
Independent Consultant
4550 North Park Ave, Apt. 505
Chevy Chase, MD 20815
Phone: (301) 654-3152
Email: Marty@hqiinc.com

Angela Drake, PhD, HMJ CTR
Site Director
Defense and Veterans Brain Injury Center

Neurology Naval Medical Center, Suite 201
San Diego, CA 92134
Phone: 619-532-5461
Email: angela.drake@med.navy.mil

Charles Engel, MD, MPH
COL, USA, MC
Associate Professor and Assistant Chair (Research)
Department of Psychiatry (USUHS)
4301 Jones Bridge Road
Bethesda, MD 20814-4799
Phone: (202)-782-8064
Email: Charles.engel@amedd.army.mil or cengel@usuhs.mil

Joseph Francis, MD, MPH
Deputy Director
Office of Quality and Performance
Department of Veterans Affairs
810 Vermont Avenue Washington, DC 20420
Phone: 202-266-4513
Email: Joe.francis@va.gov

Rosalie Fishman, RN, MSN, CPHQ President
Healthcare Quality Informatics, Inc.
15200 Shady Grove Rd, Suite 350 Rockville,
MD 20850
Phone: (301) 296-4542
Email Rosalie@hqiinc.com

Louis M. French, PsyD.
Director, Traumatic Brain Injury Service
Walter Reed Army Medical Center
Site Director, Defense and Veterans Brain Injury Center
Walter Reed Army Medical Center
6900 Georgia Ave. Bldg 1
Washington, DC 20812
Phone: 202-782-3252
Email: Louis.French@us.army.mil

Lori Simmers Geckle USACHPPM
Senior Health Risk Communicator Specialist
US Army Center for Health Promotion and Preventive Medicine
Address: 5158 Blackhawk Rd, MCHB-TS-RHR
APG MD 21010-5401; Phone: 410-436-7709
Email: lori.geckle@us.army.mil

Kathy Helmick, MS, CNRN, CRNP
Deputy Director Defense and Veterans Brain Injury Center
Walter Reed Army Medical Center
6900 Georgia Ave. Bldg 1
Washington, DC 20812
Phone:202-782-3252
Fax: 202-782-4400
Email: Katherine.helmick@amedd.army.mil

Charles Hoge, MD
COL, MC, USA
Director, Division of Psychiatry and Neuroscience
Walter Reed Army Institute of Research
503 Robert Grant Ave
Washington, DC 20307-5001
Phone: 301-319-9342
Email:charles.hoge@us.army.mil

Richard Hunt, MD
Director, Division of Injury Response
Centers for Disease Control and Prevention
1600 Clifton Rd
Atlanta, GA 30333
Phone: (770) 488-4031
Email: rhunt@cdc.gov

Robin Hurley, MD
Associate Chief of Staff, Mental Health and
MIRECC Associate Director
Salisbury, VA medical Center
601 Brenner
Salisbury, NC 28144
Phone: 704-638-3450
Email: Robin.hurley@va.gov

Michael Jaffee, MD
COL, MC, USAF, FS
National Director,
Defense and Veterans Brain Injury Center
Walter Reed Army Medical Center
6900 Georgia Ave. Bldg 1
Washington, DC 20012
Phone: 202-782-6345
Email: michael.jaffee@amedd.army.mil

Angela Klar, RN, MSN, ANP-CS
Chronic Disease Clinical Practice Guideline Coordinator
US Army Medical Command
Quality Management, Office of Evidence-Based Practice
2050 Worth Road, Bldg 2792, Suite 26
FT. Sam Houston, TX 78234
Phone: 210-221-8740(DSN 471)
Email: Angela.Klar@amedd.army.mil

Joanne E. Ksionsky, BSN
Clinical Practice Guideline Coordinator
US Army Medical Command
Quality Management, Office of Evidence-Based Practice
2050 Worth Road, Bldg 2792, Suite 26
FT. Sam Houston, TX 78234
Phone: 210 2217281
Email: Joanne.Ksionsky@amedd.army.mil

Robert Labutta, MD
COL, MC, USA
TBI Senior Executive
Defense Center of Excellence (DCoE)
for Psychological Health (PH) and Traumatic Brain Injury (TBI)
1401 Wilson Blvd, Suite 400
Arlington, VA 22209
Phone:703-696-9460
Email: Robert.labutta@us.army.mil or

Robert.labutta@ha.osd.mil
Geoffrey Ling, MD, PhD
COL, MC, USA
Professor and Vice Chair of Neurology
Department of Neurology
Uniformed Services University
4301 Jones Bridge RD
Bethesda, MD 20814
Phone: 301-295-3643
Email: gling@usuhs.mil

Lynne Lowe, PT, DPT, OCS
LTC, USA, Chief, Operations Branch/Clinical Staff Officer
Proponrncy Office for Rehabilitation and Reintegration
Health Policy and Services Office of The Surgeon General
5109 Leesburg Pike
Falls Church, VA 22041
Phone: 703-681-9997

Blackberry: 703-981-7294
Email: Lynne.Lowe@amedd.army.mil

Joanne Marko, MS, SLP
Independent Consultant
17816 Whimsey Court
Olney, MD 20832
Phone: (301) 774-5812
Email: joannemarko@gmail.com

Sheryl Mims, RN
Mild Traumatic Brain Injury Case Manager
Carl R. Darnell Army Medical Center (Clinic)
42003 Battallion Ave
Fort Hood, TX 76544
Phone:254 2888430
Email: Sheryl.Mims@amedd.army.mil

Lisa Newman, ScD
Chief, Speech Pathology Department
Research Speech Pathologist
Walter Reed Army Medical Center
Department of Surgery
Army Audiology and Speech Center
6900 Georgia Ave.
Washington, DC 20812
Phone: 202-782-8553
Email: Lisa.newman@amedd.army.mil

David T. Orman, MD, DAC
COL, MC, USA
Chief, PTSD-TBI/BH
Integration (PTBI)
HQ MEDCOM
402 Evans Ave
Alamo Heights, TX 78209
Phone: 210-221-6792
Email: david.orman@amedd.army.mil

Michelle Peterson, DPT, NCS Physical Therapist
Minneapolis VA Medical Center One Veterans Drive
Minneapolis, MN 55417
Phone: 612-467-1369
Email: michelle.peterson@va.gov

Micaela Cornis-Pop, Ph.D, SLP
Rehabilitation Planning Specialist
PM&R National Program Office
Hunter Holmes McGuire VA Medical Center
1201 Broad Rock Boulevard
Richmond, VA 23249
Phone: 804-675-5046
Email: micaela.cornispop@va.gov

Mary Ramos, RN, PhD
Medical Management Coordinator
US Army Medical Command
2050 Worth Road, Suite 26
Fort Sam Houston, TX 78234
Phone: 210-221-7281
Email: mary.ramos4@amedd.army.mil

Patricia A. Rikli, Ph.D, MSN, BSN
Project Manager/Nurse Planner
VA Employee Education System
1 Jefferson Barracks Drive
St. Louis, MO 63125-4199
Phone: (314) 894-5742
Email: patricia.rikli@va.gov

Robert L. Ruff, MD, PhD Neurology Director
Cleveland VA Medical Center 10701 East Blvd
Cleveland, OH 44106
Phone: 216-791-3800x5230
Email: robert.ruff1@va.gov

Aaron Schneiderman, PhD, MPH, RN
VHA, DC VA Medical Center
War Related Illness and Injury Study Center
50 Irving Street, NW
Washington, DC 20422
Phone: 202-745-8000 ext 6236
Email: aaron.schneiderman@va.gov

Steven G. Scott, DO
Chief, Physical Medicine and Rehabilitation
James A. Haley VA Medical Center
13000 Bruce B. Downs Blvd
Tampa, FL 33612
Phone: 813-972-7506
Email: steven.scott@va.gov

Barbara J. Sigford, MD, PhD
VHA National Director, Physical Medicine and Rehabilitation
Minneapolis VA Medical Center
1 Veterans Drive
Minneapolis, MN 55416
Phone: 612-725-2044
Email: Barbara.sigford@va.gov

Kristin A. Silva, RNC, MN, NP VA
Maryland Healthcare System Primary Care
10 North Greene Street
Baltimore, MD 21201
Phone: 410-605-7000 ext. 4841 Fax: 410-605-7873
Email: Kristin.silva@va.gov

Benjamin E. Solomon, MD
LTC, MC, USA
Chief, Neurology Service
Traumatic Brain Injury and Neurology Rehabilitation Center
Womack Army Medical Center
4-2817 Reilly RD
Ft. Bragg, NC 28310
Phone: 910-907-8019
Email: Benjamin.solomon@us.army.mil

Gretchen C. Stephens, BS, MPA, OTR/L
VHA National TBI Program Coordinator
Hunter Holmes McGuire VA Medical Center
1201 Broad Rock Boulevard
Richmond, VA 23249
Phone: 804-675-5597
Email: Gretchen.stephens@va.gov

Jay M. Stone, PhD
Lt Col, OASD (HA)/TMA
Director, Psychological Health Clinical Standards of
Care Defense Centers of Excellence for Psychological
Health and Traumatic Brain Injury
1401 Wilson Blvd Ste 400
Arlington, VA 22209
Phone: 703 696-9460 (office) or 703 507-9607 (cell)
Email: jay.Stone@tma.osd.mil

Oded Susskind, MPH
Medical Education Consultant
P.O. Bo 112

Brookline MA 02446 Phone: 617- 232-3558
Email: Oded@tiac.net

Heidi P. Terrio, MD, MPH
COL, MC, USA
Chief, Deployment Health, Fort Carson
Evans Army Community Hospital
6055 Hardwick Drive
Colorado Springs, Co
Phone: 719-524-4669
Email: heidi.terrio@amedd.army.mil

Kimialeesha Thomas, RN, MSN
Mild Traumatic Brain Injury Clinic
Ft. Hood
Bldg 42004 Battalion Ave
Fort Hood, TX 76544
Phone: 254-287-2405
Email:Kimialeesha.Thomas@amedd.army.mil

Mary Tolbert, PA-C
Clinical Coordinator-HJF Center for Defense and
Veteran's Brain Injury Center (DVBIC)
Medical Director Traumatic Brain Injury Clinic WAMC-Neurology
Fort Bragg, NC 28310
Phone: 910-907-9515
Email: marysusan.tolbert@us.army.mil

Kathryn Tortorice, Pharm D, BCPS
Clinical Pharmacy Specialist
Department of Veterans Affairs
VACO Pharmacy Benefits Management Services
1st Avenue- 1 Block North of Cermak Rd.
Building 37 Room 139
Hines, Il 60141
Phone: 708-786-7873
Email: Kathy.tortorice@va.gov

Rodney D. Vanderploeg, PhD, ABPP-CN
Clinical Neuropsychologist
James A. Haley VA Medical Center
13000 Bruce B. Downs Blvd
Tampa, FL 33612
Phone: 813-972-2000x6728
Email: Rodney.vanderploeg@va.gov

Christopher S. Williams, MD
COL, USAF, MC
SFS Senior Executive Director, Traumatic
Brain Injury Defense Centers of Excellence (DCOE) for
Psychological Health and Traumatic Brain Injury
1401 Wilson Blvd, Suite 400
Arlington, VA 22209
Phone: 703-696-9460
Email: christopher.williams2@tma.osd.mil

Warren Withlock, MD
Primary Care, OEF/OIF Post-Combat Care,
Program Director Uptown Division,
Charlie Norwood VAMC
1 Freedom Way
Augusta, GA
Phone: 706 733-0188 ext 5835
Email: Warren.Whitlock@va.gov

Appendix I: Bibliography

ACRM . American Congress of Rehabilitation Medicine Mild Traumatic Brain Injury Committee of the Head Injury Interdisciplinary Special Interest Group. Definition of mild traumatic brain injury. *J Head Trauma Rehabil* 1993;8(3):86–7.

Alves W, Macciocchi SN, Barth JT. Postconcussive symptoms after uncomplicated mild head injury. *J Head Trauma Rehabil Sept* 1993;8(3):48–59.

American Psychiatric Association. Diagnostic and statistical manual of mental disorders DSM-IV-TR (Fourth ed.). Washington D.C.: *American Psychiatric Association,* 2007.

Anonymous. Practice parameter: the management of concussion in sports (summary statement). *Report of the Quality Standards Subcommittee.* Neurology March 1997;48(3):581–5.

Ashman TA, Schwartz ME, Cantor JB, Hibbard MR, Gordon WA. Screening for substance abuse in individuals with traumatic brain injury. *Brain Inj* 2004 Feb;18(2):191-202.

Anson K, Ponsford J. Evaluation of a coping skills group following traumatic brain injury. *Brain Inj* 2006 Feb;20(2):167-78.

Bazarian JJ, Atabaki S. Predicting postconcussion syndrome after minor traumatic brain injury. *Acad Emerg Med* 2001 Aug;8(8):788-95.

Bazarian JJ, Zemlan FP, Mookerjee S, Stigbrand T. Serum S-100B and cleaved-tau are poor predictors of long-term outcome after mild traumatic brain injury. *Brain Inj* 2006 Jun;20(7):759-65.

Bazarian JJ, Beck C, Blyth B, von Ahsen N, Hasselblatt M. Impact of creatine kinase correction on the predictive value of S-100B after mild traumatic brain injury. *Restor Neurol Neurosci* 2006;24(3):163- 72.

Bédard M, Felteau M, Mazmanian D, Fedyk K, Klein R, Richardson J, Parkinson W, Minthorn-Biggs MB. Pilot evaluation of a mindfulness-based intervention to improve quality of life among individuals who sustained traumatic brain injuries. *Disabil Rehabil* 2003 Jul;25(13):722-31.

Belanger HG, Curtiss G, Demery JA, Lebowitz BK, Vanderploeg RD. Factors moderating neuropsychological outcomes following mild traumatic brain injury: a meta-analysis. *J Int Neuropsychol Soc* 2005 May;11(3):215–27.

Belanger HG, Vanderploeg RD. The neuropsychological impact of sports-related concussion: a meta-analysis. *J Int Neuropsychol Soc* 2005 Jul;11(4):345–57.

Bianchini KJ, Curtis KL, Greve KW. Compensation and malingering in traumatic brain injury: a dose-response relationship? *Clin Neuropsychol* 2006 Dec;20(4):831-47.

Biberthaler P, Mussack T, Wiedemann E, Kanz KG, Koelsch M, Gippner-Steppert C, Jochum M. Evaluation of S-100b as a specific marker for neuronal damage due to minor head trauma. *World J Surg* 2001 Jan;25(1):93-7.

Bigler ED, Blatter DD, Johnson SC, Anderson CV, Russo AA, Gale SD, Ryser DK, MacNamara SE, Bailey BJ. Traumatic brain injury, alcohol and quantitative neuro imaging: preliminary findings. *Brain Inj* 1996 Mar;10(3):197-206.

Binder L, Rohling M. Money matters: a meta-analytic review of the effects of financial incentives on recovery after closed-head injury. *Am J Psychiatry* 1996 Jan;153(1):7–10.

Binder LM, Rohling ML, Larrabee, GJ. A review of mild head trauma, Part I: Meta-analytic review of neuropsychological studies. *J Clin Exp Neuropsychol* 1997 June; 19(3):421–31.

Boake C, McCauley SR, Levin HS, Contant CF, Song JX, Brown SA, Goodman HS, Brundage SI, DiazMarchan PJ, Merritt SG. Limited agreement between criteria-based diagnoses of postconcussional syndrome. *J Neuropsychiatry Clin Neurosci* 2004 Fall;16(4):493-9.

Boake C, McCauley SR, Levin HS, Pedroza C, Contant CF, Song JX, Brown SA, Goodman H, Brundage SI, Diaz-Marchan PJ. Diagnostic criteria for postconcussional syndrome after mild to moderate traumatic brain injury. *J Neuropsychiatry Clin Neurosci* 2005 Summer;17(3):50-6.

Bombardier CH, Temkin NR, Machamer J, Dikmen SS. The natural history of drinking and alcohol-related problems after traumatic brain injury. *Arch Phys Med Rehabil* 2003 Feb:84(2):185-91.

Borg J, Holm L, Peloso PM, Cassidy JD, Carroll LJ, von Holst H, Paniak C, Yates D; WHO Collaborating Centre Task Force on Mild Traumatic Brain Injury. Non-surgical intervention and cost for mild traumatic brain injury: results of the WHO Collaborating Centre Task Force on mild traumatic brain injury. *J Rehabil Med* 2004 Feb; (43 Suppl):76-83.

Broshek DK, Kaushik T, Freeman JR, Erlanger D, Webbe F, Barth JT. Sex differences in outcome following sports-related concussion. *J Neurosurg* 2005 May;102(5):856-63.

Bryant RA, Moulds MM, Guthrie R, Nixon RD . Treating acute stress disorder following mild traumatic brain injury. *Am J Psychiatry* 2003 Mar;160(3):585-7.

Catena RD, van Donkelaar P, Chou LS. Cognitive task effects on gait stability following concussion. *Exp Brain Res* 2007 Jan;176(1):23-31.

Cantu RC. Guidelines for return to contact sports after a cerebral concussion. *Physician Sports Med* 1986;14(10):76–9.

Cantu RC. Return to play guidelines after a head injury. *Clin Sports Med* 1998 Jan;17(1): 45–60.

Carroll LJ, Cassidy JD, Peloso PM, Borg J, von Holst H, Holm L, Paniak C, Pépin M; WHO Collaborating Centre Task Force on Mild Traumatic Brain Injury. Prognosis for mild traumatic brain injury: results of the WHO collaborating centre task force on mild traumatic brain injury. *J Rehab Med* 2004 Feb;36(43 Suppl):84–105.

Cassidy JD, Carroll LJ, Peloso PM, Borg J, von Holst H, Holm L, Kraus J, Coronado VG. Incidence, risk factors and prevention of mild traumatic brain injury: results of the WHO collaboration centre task force on mild traumatic brain injury. *J Rehabil Med* 2004 Feb: (43 Suppl):28–60.

Chamelian L, Feinstein A. Outcome after mild to moderate traumatic brain injury: the role of dizziness. *Arch Phys Med Rehabil* 2004 Oct;85(10):1662-6.

Chaput G, Lavigne G, Paquet J, Manzini C, Giguère J, Demers A, Denis R. Time course prevalence of sleep disturbances and mood alterations after mild traumatic brain injury: a preliminary report. *Sleep* 2007;30:A302-A3.

Cicerone KD. Remediation of 'working attention' in mild traumatic brain injury. *Brain Inj* 2002 Mar; 16(3): 185-95.

Cicerone KD, Dahlberg C, Malec JF, Langenbahn DM, Felicetti T, Kneipp S, Ellmo W, Kalmar K, Giacino JT, Harley JP, Laatsch L, Morse PA, Catanese J. Evidence-based cognitive rehabilitation: updated review of the literature from 1998 through 2002. *Arch Phys Med Rehabil* 2005 Aug;86(8): 1681-92.

Colligan SC, Tellier JE, Campbell CA, Adey G, Chen T, Gaub K, Taekman H, Tellier J, Wolcott C, Yee R. Predictors of functional outcome in mild traumatic brain injury. *Clin Neuropsychol* 2005;19:540.

Committee on Gulf War and Health: Brain Injury in Veterans and Long-term outcomes. Institute of Medicine, Washington DC. Gulf War and Health, Volume 7: *Long-term Consequences of Traumatic Brain Injury*. Washington, DC: The National Academies Press; 2008. 396 p.

Comper P, Bissghop S M, Garnide N, Triggo A. A systematic review of treatments for mild traumatic brain injury. *Brain Inj* 2005 Oct;19(11):863-80.

Dawson KS, Batchelor J, Meares S, Chapman J, Marosszeky JE. Applicability of neural reserve theory in mild traumatic brain injury. *Brain Inj* 2007 Aug;21(9):943-9.

Deb S, Lyons I, Koutzoukis C. Neurobehavioural symptoms one year after a head injury. *B B J Psychiatry* 1999 Apr;174:360–5.

DeHaan A, Halterman C, Langan J, Drew AS, Osternig LR, Chou LS, van Donkelaar P. Cancelling planned actions following mild traumatic brain injury. *Neuropsychologia* 2007 Jan;45(2):406-11.

de Kruijk JR, Leffers P, Menheere PP, Meerhoff S, Rutten J, Twijnstra A. Prediction of post-traumatic complaints after mild traumatic brain injury: early symptoms and biochemical markers. *J Neurol Neurosurg Psychiatry* 2002 Dec;73(6):727-32.

Dikmen S, McLean A, Temkin N. Neuropsychological and psychosocial consequences of minor head injury. *J Neurol Neurosurg Psychiatry* 1986;49(11):1227–32.

Dikmen SS, Bombardier CH, Machamer JE, Fann JR, Temkin NR. Natural history of depression in traumatic brain injury. *Arch Phys Med Rehabil* 2004 Sep;85(9):1457-64.

Dirette DK, Plaisier BR. The development of self-awareness of deficits from 1 week to 1 year after traumatic brain injury: preliminary findings. *Brain Inj* 2007 Oct;21(11):1131-6.

Ernst A, Basta D, Seidl RO, Todt I, Scherer H, Clarke A. Management of posttraumatic vertigo. *Otolaryngol Head Neck Surg* 2005 Apr;132(4):554-8.

Evered L, Ruff R, Baldo J, Isomura A. Emotional risk factors and postconcussional disorder. *Assessment* 2003 Dec;1094):420-7.

Fann JR, Burington B, Leonetti A, Jaffe K, Katon WJ, Thompson RS. Psychiatric illness following traumatic brain injury in an adult health maintenance organization population. *Arch Gen Psychiatry* 2004 Jan;61(1):53-61.

Ghaffar O, McCullagh S, Ouchterlony D, Feinstein A. Randomized treatment trial in mild traumatic brain injury. *J Psychosom Res* 2006 Aug;61(2):153-60.

Gilworth G, Eyres S, Carey A, Bhakta BB, Tennant A. Working with a brain injury: personal experiences of returning to work following a mild or moderate brain injury. *J Rehabil Med* 2008 May;40(5):334-9.

Gotshall KR, Gray NL, Drake AI, Tejidor R Hoffer ME, McDonald EC. To investigate the influence of acute vestibular impairment following mild traumatic brain injury on subsequent ability to remain on active duty 12 months later. *Military Medicine* 2007 Aug;172:852-7.

Gunstad J, Suhr JA. "Expectation as etiology" versus "the good old days": postconcussion syndrome symptom reporting in athletes, headache sufferers, and depressed individuals. *J Int Neuropsychol Soc* 2001 Mar;7(3):323-3.

Guskiewicz KM, McCrea M, Marshall SW, Cantu RC, Randolph C, Barr W, Onate JA, Kelly JP. Cumulative effects associated with recurrent concussion in collegiate football players: the NCAA Concussion Study. *JAMA* 2003 Nov 19;290(19):2549-55.

Guskiewicz KM, Marshall SW, Bailes J, McCrea M, Cantu RC, Randolph C, Jordan BD. Association between recurrent concussion and late-life cognitive impairment in retired professional football players. *Neurosurgery* 2005 Oct;57(4):719-26.

Halterman CI, Langan J, Drew A, Rodriguez E, Osternig LR, Chou LS, van Donkelaar P. Tracking the recovery of visuospatial attention deficits in mild traumatic brain injury. *Brain* 2006 Mar;129(Pt 3):747-53.

Hartlage LC, Durant-Wilson D, Patch PC. Persistent neurobehavioral problems following mild traumatic brain injury. *Arch Clin Neuropsychol* 2001 Aug; 16(6):561–70.

Hibbard MR, Cantor J, Charatz H, Rosenthal R, Ashman T, Gundersen N, Ireland-Knight L, Gordon W, Avner J, Gartner A. Peer support in the community: initial findings of a mentoring program for individuals with traumatic brain injury and their families. *J Head Trauma Rehabil* 2002 Apr;17(2):112- 31.

Heitger MH, Jones RD, Dalrymple-Alford JC, Frampton CM, Ardagh MW, Anderson TJ. Motor deficits and recovery during the first year following mild closed head injury. *Brain Inj* 2006 Jul;20(8):807-24.

Heitger MH, Anderson TJ, Jones RD, Dalrymple-Alford JC, Frampton CM, Ardagh MW. Eye movement and visuomotor arm movement deficits following mild closed head injury. *Brain* 2004 Mar;127(Pt 3):575- 90.

Hinkle JL, Alves WM, Rimell RW, Jane JA. Restoring social competence in minor head-injury patients. *J Neurosci Nurs* 1986 Oct;18(5):268-71.

Hoffer ME, Gottshall KR, Moore R, Balough BJ, Wester D. Characterizing and treating dizziness after mild head trauma. *Otol Neurotol* 2004 Mar;25(2):135-8.

Hoge CW, McGurk D, Thomas J, Cox A, Engel C, Castro CA. Mild traumatic brain injury in U.S. soldiers returning from Iraq. *N Engl J Med* 2008 Jan 31;358(5):455-63.

Holm L, Cassidy JD, Carroll LJ, Borg Jr. Summary of the WHO collaborating centre for neurotrauma task force on mild traumatic brain injury. *J Rehabil Med* 2005 May;37(3):137-41.

Horner MD, Ferguson PL, Selassie AW, Labbate LA, Kniele K, Corrigan JD. Patterns of alcohol use 1 year after traumatic brain injury: a population-based, epidemiological study. *J Int Neuropsychol Soc* 2005 May;11(3):322-30.

Iverson GL, Brooks BL, Lovell MR, Collins MW. No cumulative effects for one or two previous concussions. *Br J Sports Med* 2006 Jan;40(1):72-5.

Iverson GL. Misdiagnosis of the persistent postconcussion syndrome in patients with depression. *Arch Clin Neuropsychol* 2006;21(4):303-10.

Iverson GL, Zasler ND, Lange RT. Post-concussive disorder. In Zasler ND, Katz DI, Zafonte RD.,editors. Brain Injury Medicine: Principles and Practice. New York, New York: 2007: *Demos Medical Publishing LLC;* 2007.

Kashluba S, Paniak C, Casey JE. Persistent symptoms associated with factors identified by the WHO Task Force on Mild Traumatic Brain Injury. *Clin Neuropsychol* 2008 Mar;22(2):195-208.

Kashluba S, Casey JE, Paniak C. Evaluating the utility of ICD-10 diagnostic criteria for postconcussion syndrome following mild traumatic brain injury. *J Int Neuropsychol Soc* 2006 Jan;12(1):111-8.

Kissick J, Johnston K. Return to play after concussion: principles and practice. *Clin J Sport Med* 2005;15(6):426-31.

Kushner D. Mild traumatic brain injury. *Arch Intern Med* 1998 Aug 10-24;158(15):1617-24.

Landre N, Poppe CJ, Davis N, Schmaus B, Hobbs SE. Cognitive functioning and postconcussive symptoms in trauma patients with and without mild TBI. *Arch Clin Neuropsychol* 2006 May;21(4):255–73.

Luis CA, Vanderploeg RD, Curtiss G. Predictors of postconcussion symptom complex in community dwelling male veterans. *J Int Neuropsychol Soc* 2003 Nov;9(7):1001-15.

Macciocchi SN, Barth JT, Alves WA, Rimel RW, Jane JA. Neuropsychological functioning and recovery following mild head injury in collegiate athletes. *Neurosurgery* 1996 Sep;39(3):510–4.

MacMillan PJ, Hart RP, Martelli MF, Zasler ND. Pre-injury status and adaptation following traumatic brain injury. *Brain Inj* 2002 Jan;16(1):41-9.

Mahmood O, Rapport LJ, Hanks RA, Fichtenberg NL. Neuropsychological Performance and Sleep Disturbance Following Traumatic Brain Injury. *J Head Trauma Rehabil* 2004 Sep-Oct;19(5):378-90.

Malec JF, Testa JA, Rush BK, Brown AW, Moessner AM. Self-assessment of impairment, impaired self-awareness, and depression after traumatic brain injury. *J Head Trauma Rehabil* 2007 MayJun;22(3):156-66.

McCauley SR, Boake C, Levin HS, Contant CF, Song JX. Postconcussional disorder following mild to moderate traumatic brain injury: anxiety, depression, and social support as risk factors and comorbidities. *J Clin Exp Neuropsychol* 2001Dec;23(6):792-808.

McCrea M, Guskiewicz KM, Marshall SW, Barr W, Randolph C, Cantu RC, Onate JA, Yang J. Kelly JP. Acute effects and recovery time following concussion in collegiate football players: the NCAA Concussion Study *JAMA* 2003 Nov 19;290(19):2556-63.

McCrea M, Kelly JP, Randolph C, Cisler R, Berger L. Immediate neurocognitive effects of concussion. *Neurosurgery* 2002 May;5095):1032-40.

Mehta KM, Ott A, Kalmijn S, Slooter AJ, van Duijn CM, Hofman A, Breteler MM. Head trauma and risk of dementia and Alzheimer's disease:The Rotterdam Study. *Neurology* 1999 Dec10;53(9):1959-62.

McAllister TW, Sparling MB, Flashman LA, Saykin AJ. Neuroimaging findings in mild traumatic brain injury. *J Clin Exp Neuropsychol* 2001;23(6):775-91.

Meares S, Shores EA, Taylor AJ, Batchelor J, Bryant RA, Baguley IJ, Chapman J, Gurka J, Dawson K, Capon L, Marosszeky JE. Mild traumatic brain injury does not predict acute postconcussion syndrome. *J Neurol Neurosurg Psychiatry* 2008 Mar;79(3):300-6.

Mittenberg W, Tremont G, Zielinski RE, Fichera S, Rayls KR. Cognitive-behavioral prevention of postconcussion syndrome. *Arch Clin Neuropsychol* 1996;11(2):139-45.

Mittenberg W, Strauman S. Diagnosis of mild head injury and the postconcussion syndrome. *J Head Trauma Rehabil* 2000 Apr;15(2):783-91.

Moldover JE, Goldberg KB, Prout MF. Depression after traumatic brain injury: A review of evidence for clinical heterogeneity. *Neuropsychol Rev* 2004 Sep;14(3):143–54.

Mooney G, Speed J. The association between mild traumatic brain injury and psychiatric conditions. *Brain Inj* 2001 Oct;15(10):865-77.

Mooney G, Speed J, Sheppard S. Factors related to recovery after mild traumatic brain injury. *Brain Inj* 2005 Nov;19(12):975-87.

Moore E L, TerryBerry-Spohr L, Hope DA. Mild traumatic brain injury and anxiety sequelae: a review of the literature. *Brain Inj* 2006 Feb;20(2):117-32.

Mussack T, Dvorak J, Graf-Baumann T, Jochum M. Serum S-100B protein levels in young amateur soccer players after controlled heading and normal exercise. *E J Med Res* 2003 Oct 22;8(10):457-64.

National Center for Injury Prevention and Control. Report to congress on mild traumatic brain injury in the United States: steps to prevent a serious public health problem. Atlanta, GA: Centers for Disease Control and Prevention;2003.

Nölle C, Todt I, Seidl RO, Ernst A. Pathophysiological changes of the central auditory pathway after blunt trauma of the head. *J Neurotrauma* 2004 Mar;21(3):251-8.

Ouellet MC, Beaulieu-Bonneau S, Morin CM. Insomnia in patients with traumatic brain injury: frequency, characteristics, and risk factors. *J Head Trauma Rehabil* 2006 May-Jun;21(3):199-212.

Pagulayan KF, Temkin NR, Machamer JE, Dikmen SS. The measurement and magnitude of awareness difficulties after traumatic brain injury: a longitudinal study. *J Int Neuropsychol Soc* 2007 Jul;13(4):561-70.

Paniak C, Toller-Lobe G, Durand A, Nagy J. A randomized trial of two treatments for mild traumatic brain injury. *Brain Inj* 1998 Dec;12(12):1011-23.

Paniak C, Toller-Lobe G, Melnyk A, Nagy J. Prediction of vocational status three to four months after treated mild traumatic brain injury. *J Musculoskel Pain* 2000;8:193-200.

Paniak C, Reynolds S, Toller-Lobe G, Melnyk A, Nagy J, Schmidt D. A longitudinal study of the relationship between financial compensation and symptoms after treated mild traumatic brain injury. *J Clin Exp Neuropsychol* 2002 Apr;24(2):187-93.

Parker TM, Osternig LR, Van Donkelaar P, Chou LS. Gait stability following concussion. *Med Sci Sports Exer* 2006 Jun;38(6):1032-40.

Parry-Jones BL, Vaughan FL, Cox, MC. Traumatic brain injury and substance misuse: a systematic review of prevalence and outcomes research (1994-2004). *Neuropsychol Rehabil* 2006 Oct;16(5):537-60.

Peloso PM, Carroll LJ, Cassidy JD, Borg J, von Holst H, Holm L, Yates D. Critical evaluation of the existing guidelines on mild traumatic brain injury. *J Rehabil Med* 2004 Feb;(43 Suppl):106-12.

Pellman EJ, Lovell MR, Viano DC, Casson IR, Tucker AM. Concussion in professional football: neuropsychological testing--part 6. *Neurosurgery* 2004 Dec;55(6):1290-303.

Ponsford J, Willmott C, Rothwell A, Cameron P, Kelly AM, Nelms R, Curran C, Ng K. Factors influencing outcome following mild traumatic brain injury in adults. *J Int Neuropsychol Soc* 2000 Jul;6(5):568-79.

Ponsford J, Willmott C, Rothwell A, Cameron P, Kelly AM, Nelms R, Curran C. Impact of early intervention on outcome following mild head injury in adults. *J Neurol Neurosurg Psychiatry* 2002 Sep;73(3):330- 2.

Ponsford J. Rehabilitation interventions after mild head injury. *Curr Opin Neurol* 2005 Dec;18(6):692-7.

Powell TJ, Collin C, Sutton K. A follow-up study of patients hospitalized after minor head injury. *Disabil Rehabil* 1996 May; 18(5):231–7.

Rapoport MJ, Feinstein A. Age and functioning after mild traumatic brain injury: the acute picture. *Brain Inj* 2001 Oct;15(10):857-64.

Rapoport MJ, McCullagh S, Streiner D, Feinstein A. The clinical significance of major depression following mild traumatic brain injury. *Psychosomatics* 2003 Jan-Feb;44(1):31-7.

Rapoport MJ, Kiss A, Feinstein A. The impact of major depression on outcome following mild- to-moderate traumatic brain injury in older adults. *J Affect Disord* 2006;92(2-3):273-6.

Reynolds S, Paniak C, Toller-Lobe G, Nagy J. A longitudinal study of compensation-seeking and return to work in a treated mild traumatic brain injury sample. *J Head Trauma Rehabil* 2003 MarApr;18(2):139-47.

Rose JM. Continuum of care model for managing mild traumatic brain injury in a workers' compensation context: a description of the model and its development. *Brain Inj* 2005 Jan;19(1):29-39.

Schretlen DJ, Shapiro AM. A quantitative review of the effects of traumatic brain injury on cognitive functioning. *Int Rev Psychiatry* 2003 Nov;15(4):341–9.

Soo C, Tate R. Psychological treatment for anxiety in people with traumatic brain injury. *Cochrane Database Syst Rev* 2007 Jul 18;(3):CD005239.

Staab JP, Ruckenstein MJ. Expanding the differential diagnosis of chronic dizziness. *Arch Otolaryngol Head Neck Surg* 2007 Feb;133(2):170-6.

Stalnacke BM, Tegner Y, Sojka P. Playing ice hockey and basketball increases serum levels of S-100B in elite players - a pilot study. *Clin J Sport Med* 2003 Sep;13(5):292-302.

Stranjalis G, Tsamandouraki K, Sakas DE, Alamanos Y. Elevated serum S-100B protein as a predictor of failure to short-term return to work or activities after mild head injury. *J Neurotrauma,* 2004 Aug; 21(8):1070-5.

Stulemeijer M, van der Werf S, Bleijenberg G, Biert J, Brauer J, Vos PE. Recovery from mild traumatic brain injury: a focus on fatigue. *J Neurol* 2006 Aug;253(8):1041-7.

Stulemeijer M, Vos PE, Bleijenberg G, van der Werf SP. Cognitive complaints after mild traumatic brain injury: Things are not always what they seem. *J Psychosoma Res* 2007 Dec;63(6):637-45.

Suh M, Kolster R, Sarkar R, McCandliss B, Ghajar J. Deficits in predictive smooth pursuit after mild traumatic brain injury. *Neurosci Lett* 2006 Jun;401(1-2):108-13.

Suhr JA, Gunstad J. Postconcussive symptom report: the relative influence of head injury and depression. *J Clin Exp Neuropsychol* 2002 Dec;24(8):981-93.

Tiersky LA, Anselmi V, Johnston MV, Kurtyka J, Roosen E, Schwartz T, Deluca J. A trial of neuropsychologic rehabilitation in mild-spectrum traumatic brain injury. *Arch Phys Med Rehabil* 2005 Aug;86(8):1565-74.

Tinius TP. The intermediate visual and auditory continuous performance test as a neuropsychological measure. *Arch Clin Neuropsychol* 2003 Mar;18(2):199-214.

Tinius TP. The Integrated Visual and Auditory Continuous Performance Test as a neuropsychological measure. *Arch Clini Neuropsychol* 2003 Jul;18(5):439-54.

Turner AP, Bombardier CH, Rimmele CT. A typology of alcohol use patterns among persons with recent traumatic brain injury or spinal cord injury: implications for treatment matching. *Arch Phys Med Rehabil* 2003 Mar;8493):358-64.

Uomoto JM, Fann JR. Explanatory style and perception of recovery in symptomatic mild traumatic brain injury. Rehabil Psychol 2004;49:334-7.

van der Naalt J. Prediction of outcome in mild to moderate head injury: a review. *J Clin Exp Neuropsychol* 2001 Dec;23(6):837-51.

Vanderploeg R D, Curtiss G, Belanger HG. Adverse long-term neuropsychological outcomes following mild traumatic brain injury. *J Inter Neuropsychol Soc* 2005;11:228-36.

Vanderploeg RD, Curtiss G, Luis CA, Salazar AM. Long-term morbidities following self-reported mild traumatic brain injury. *J Clin Exp Neuropsychol* 2007 Aug;29(6):585-98.

Wade DT, Crawford S, Wenden FJ, King NS, Moss NE. Does routine follow up after head injury help? A randomised controlled trial. *J Neurol Neurosurg Psychiatry* 1997 May;62(5):478-84.

Wade DT, King NS, Wenden FJ, Crawford S, Caldwell FE. Routine follow up after head injury: a second randomised controlled trial. *J Neurol Neurosurg Psychiatry* 1998 Aug;65(2):177-83.

World health Organization, editors. International Statistical Classification of Diseases and Related Health Problems. 10 th ed. American Psychiatric Publishing; Arlington, Virginia , 1992. 1244p.

Wood RL. Understanding the 'miserable minority': a diasthesis-stress paradigm for post-concussional syndrome. *Brain Inj* 2004 Nov;18(11):1135-53.

Wang Y, Chan RC, Deng Y. Examination of postconcussion-like symptoms in healthy university students: relationships to subjective and objective neuropsychological function performance. *Arch Clin Neuropsychol* 2006 May;21(4):339-47.

Yang CC, Tu YK, Hua MS, Huang SJ. The association between the postconcussion symptoms and clinical outcomes for patients with mild traumatic brain injury. *J Trauma* 2007 Mar;62(3):657-63.

Zasler ND, Katz DI, Zafonte RD. Mild TBI. Brain injury medicine: principles and practice. Zasler ND, Katz DI, Zafonte RD.,editors, New York, New York: Demos Medical Publishing LLC, 2007.

Ziino C, Ponsford J. Measurement and prediction of subjective fatigue following traumatic brain injury. *J Int Neuropsychol Soc* 2005 Jul;11(4):416-25.

INDEX

B

C

D

H

I

N

O

P

Q

R

W

Y